UNDERSTANDING THE PATHWAY OF PREGNANCY.

Exploring the uncommon ways,Investigating Wellbeing , Feelings, Advancement, Nourishment, Mental Prosperity, Breastfeeding, and Taking care of oneself During Your Pregnancy Process.

By

Mikayla Edgell

COPYRIGHT

Disclaimer:

The information provided on this platform is for general informational purposes only. It is not intended as medical, legal, or professional advice. Mikayla Edgell does not assume any responsibility for the accuracy, completeness, or usefulness of the information provided. Any reliance you place on such information is strictly at your own risk.

Before making decisions based on the information provided, we recommend consulting with qualified professionals in the relevant field. Mikayla Edgell is not liable for any losses, injuries, or damages arising from the use of this information

About The Author

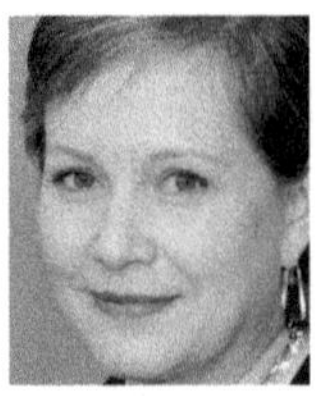

Hello, lovely readers. I am Mikayla Edgell and i am over the
Moon to share a bit about myself. While i claim to be a
superwoman , i am passionate about all things related to
Pregnancy and motherhood.
Who Am I?
In essence , i am just someone who has been on the
pregnancy
Journey and want to lend a helping hand to fellow
moms-to-be

I am here to share practical insight and emotional support in
The uniqueness of pregnancy.

Why This Book?
It is my heart poured out on every page, with the aim of making
The journey smooth . From understanding the early signs, to
What happens weekly, to embracing emotions and ensuring
Your mental health is sound. Hey this book is simply saying
You've got this.

Cheers to you and the awesome journey ahead.

Start of Something New!

INTRODUCTION

Hello, future moms! Welcome to "UNDERSTANDING THE PATHWAY OF PREGNANCY."

Our goal is to be your trusted companion as you embark on this magical adventure. Throughout this guide, we will help you understand the signs of a healthy pregnancy and support you through the ups and downs of your emotions. Together, we will explore the incredible development of your baby, from the first flutters to the joyous arrival. We will also discuss the importance of a nutritious diet for both you and your little one. And let's not forget the importance of self-care during this transformative time. So sit back, relax, and let's make these upcoming months the most memorable of your life!

CHAPTER ONE

Knowing The Fundamentals Of Conception And Fertility

Sperms are ejaculated into the woman's vagina during sexual activity. After passing through the cervix and the uterus, the sperm eventually arrives at the fallopian tubes, where fertilisation can take place. Fertilisation occurs when a sperm reaches the egg effectively. The fertilised egg passes through numerous stages of development after fertilisation. It first develops into an embryo, which inserts itself into the uterine lining.After that, it keeps growing and changing, eventually becoming a foetus and then a baby. The seamless harmony with which these systems operate is simply amazing. It is just astounding how much coordination and precision are needed at the microscopic level. Considering how complicated everything is, it makes sense that occasionally things might not go as planned.

A Portion of the sperm that enters a woman's vagina during ovulation may pass via her cervix and uterus before arriving at her Fallopian tube. One sperm is supposed to successfully reach the egg and fertilise it. Fertilisation generally takes place in a day or two. The fertilised egg, called a zygote, starts to resolve after fertilisation. It divides constantly, dividing first into two cells, also into four, and so on. The end result of this division process is the creation of an embryo. The embryo leaves the Fallopian tube after about two to three days and begins to travel towards the uterus, occasionally pertaining to the womb. The embryo will start to cleave to the uterine wall if the filling of the uterus is acceptable for implantation, which is generally the case during this stage of a woman's menstrual cycle. **Implantation** is the term for this attaching procedure, which generally takes place five days following ovulation.

The embryo is known as a blastocyst at this point.The placenta, an element of the growing embryo, starts to make the hormone hCG(mortal chorionic gonadotropin) as implantation progresses. This hormone is essential for maintaining the gestation. It forms the foundation of a gestation test and is discharged into the woman's blood and urine. Because of the presence of hCG hormone, a positive gestation test result can generally be achieved 10 to

16 days following ovulation.The couple must have sexual relations both before and during the woman's ovulation phase for all of the forenamed to be. There will not be another occasion for the sperm to fertilise an egg other than now. Couples that engage in frequent and vigorous sexual exertion, frequently having coitus every two to three days, do not have to worry about a particular" rich time." There will be plenty of sexual action between them. In the ovaries, eggs — also pertaining to as ova or oocytes are kept in bitsy sacs called follicles.

An ultrasound checkup can be used to view these follicles. From birth, women have all of their eggs in their ovaries. One to two million eggs, halted in their early development stage, are present in their ovaries at birth. Several eggs begin to develop each month as women approach puberty, but only one or two are released during ovulation. The ultimate step of an egg's development happens only after a sperm fertilizes it. The egg is an amazing cell that's visible to the unaided eye and is surprisingly huge for a mortal body cell. Like sperm, eggs have half of the normal number of chromosomes in their capitals, which is twenty- three.

These chromosomes combine with the 23 manly chromosomes during fertilisation to induce a completely developed fertilised egg with 46 chromosomes overall. The egg not only includes chromosomes but also essential factors like mitochondria, which are in charge of producing energy for the cell. Unexpectedly, the egg, not the sperm, controls and determines the first three days of an embryo's life. Your healthcare provider at this point focuses on what you can do to increase your chances of having a healthy baby .It's possible that you have also considered how to achieve these objectives.

For example, you used a safe system of birth control when you did not want a child.It's pivotal to take action to reach your goal of getting pregnant and giving birth to a healthy child now that you are considering getting pregnant!

These Conduct Comprise Of The Following

1.Before deciding to become pregnant, make sure you discuss your options with your doctor,your health and any current medical conditions that may have an impact on your baby should be discussed with your doctor. In addition, they may want to talk about any issues you had with previous gravities, current specifics, any immunisations you may bear, and preventive measures you can take ahead of getting pregnant to lower your chance of certain birth abnormalities.

2. Taking into account individual preferences and points for conserving the health of the expectant mama and her future child. ensure that you get 400 micrograms of folic acid daily. One form of B vitamin that's vital to your body is folic acid. Having acceptable folic acid in your system is veritably important both one month before and during gestation. This is due to the fact that folic acid, which can help prevent disastrous birth scars in the baby's brain and spine , similar to anencephaly, is recommended for all individuals who are able to get pregnant. This can be fulfilled by taking supplements, eating healthy, fortified with nutrients.It's also critical to have a balanced diet full of foods high in folate.

3. Our health can be harmed by dangerous chemicals, man made substances, certain metals,

insect repellents, fertilisers, and even animal waste like cat or rat faeces. These may negatively affect a person's reproductive system, which may make it more difficult for them to become pregnant. Exposure during pregnancy, infancy, childhood, or puberty, even in little levels, can raise the chance of getting certain disorders. In both our homes and workplaces, it is critical that we educate ourselves on the best ways to safeguard our loved ones and ourselves from these dangerous chemicals.

4. For everyone, achieving and sustaining a healthy weight is crucial. Obesity and excess weight exposes the risk of major illnesses like heart disease, type 2 diabetes, and several types of cancer. In a similar vein, being underweight can also have negative health effects. It takes more than brief dietary adjustments to reach and maintain a healthy weight. It involves embracing a way of life that involves regular physical activity and a balanced diet. Before deciding to become pregnant, it is advisable to speak with your doctor about methods for achieving and maintaining a healthy weight if you are underweight, overweight, or obese.

5. You can learn vital information that could affect your baby's early development or your own chances of becoming pregnant by researching your family's medical history. It's likely that you are unaware of the potential effects that your cousin's sickle cell illness or your sister's heart defect could have on your unborn child, but it is important to let your doctor know about this family history. In light of your family's medical history, your physician might suggest genetic counselling. In cases of multiple miscarriages, infant deaths, infertility problems, or if you have already encountered a genetic disorder or birth defect during a pregnancy, genetic counselling is also recommended.

6.Mental well-being encompasses our attitudes, feelings, and actions as we move through life. It's critical to have self-worth and a good view on life in order to be at our best. Periodically feeling stressed, depressed, anxious, or worried is normal. You must, however, get help if these feelings continue to interfere with your daily tasks. Discuss your feelings and the various treatment options with your healthcare professional.

Learning About Pregnancy

A person may experience a number of feelings upon learning they are pregnant, including happiness and excitement as well as surprise, confusion, and distress. Every person has a different experience on this journey.

Your hormone levels can fluctuate, which can amplify your emotions and contribute to these emotional swings. Sharing your worries and anxieties with someone else might help you feel supported and at ease

Actions to Take Following the Discovery of Pregnancy

See A Medical Practitioner

A Medical practitioner will use an early ultrasound or blood test to confirm your pregnancy at this visit. To guarantee a safe start to your pregnancy, they will also go over your medical history and any drugs you may be taking. They will also determine your due date and give you a wealth of information on what to expect from your pregnancy. Please feel free to ask any questions you may have of your pregnancy care provider; jotting them down in advance can ensure you don't forget them. Take prenatal vitamins beginning now, if you haven't already, you should start taking prenatal vitamins. The vitamins and minerals required for a healthy pregnancy are provided by these vitamins. Folate is an essential vitamin that helps lower the risk of neural tube abnormalities, which can result in spina bifida. Prenatal vitamins should include calcium, magnesium, zinc, copper, vitamin B12, and vitamins A, C, D, and E in addition to folate. Additionally, your physician could advise taking an iron supplement on its own. Recent study indicates that choline—which is crucial for placental and brain development—may be included in some prenatal supplements. Docosahexaenoic acid (DHA), which is crucial for the development and operation of your baby's brain, may also be present in them.

Be Sure To Discuss Any Medications Or Supplements You Are Currently Taking With Your Doctor Or Other Pregnancy Care Provider.

Due to their potential to cross the placenta, not all drugs and supplements are safe to use while pregnant. It is equally crucial, though, to continue taking all of your prescriptions as prescribed by your physician. Severe negative effects can occur when some drugs, including antidepressants, are stopped suddenly. Your healthcare provider can help you develop a plan to progressively cut back on the usage of drugs that are not advised to be taken while pregnant. It is best to avoid using some painkillers, such as ibuprofen (Advil or Motrin), when pregnant. You can find out which over-the-counter drugs are safe to consume from your healthcare professional.

For example, you can safely take paracetamol (Tylenol) if you have a fever or headache while pregnant. There are certain over-the-counter drugs that you can take if you have allergies.To guarantee your baby's safety as well as your own, it is advisable to speak with your doctor and get personalized recommendations.

Make A Work Plan.

Until you are ready, you are not required to tell your employer that you are pregnant. But scheduling time for doctor's visits and creating a backup plan in case something goes wrong are crucial. Make sure you are also well-versed in the maternity policies of both your employer and state.

Reducing Your Caffeine Intake Is Advised To Ensure A Safe Pregnancy.

This is due to the fact that caffeine can cross the placenta and is metabolized more slowly in pregnant women. It is advised to keep your daily caffeine consumption to 200 mg or less, or around two cups of normal coffee. Additionally, research has shown that ingesting more than 200 mg of caffeine daily raises the possibility of miscarriage. It's critical to keep an eye on how much caffeine you consume from all sources, including tea, soda, and dark chocolate.

Pay Close Attention To Your Diet, Particularly If You're Expecting.

To grow and thrive, your baby requires the proper amount of nutrients. Drink plenty of water and consume well-balanced meals rich in fiber, protein, healthy fats, complex carbohydrates, and vitamins and minerals. Good options include fruits, vegetables, whole grains, legumes, dairy, and cooked lean meats. But because they can be dangerous, there are several foods you should avoid when pregnant. High mercury seafood, such as swordfish and huge tuna, sushi, raw or undercooked meat, fish, and eggs, raw sprouts, unwashed produce, unpasteurized milk, cheese, and fruit juice, and deli meat are some examples of these. Don't forget to thoroughly cook all the fish and meats.

MY PREGNANCY JOURNEY AND ME

CHAPTER TWO

Relating The First Pointers Of Gestation.

Knowing the early signs of gestation is pivotal to understanding what your body is going through. The following are typical pointers to be apprehensive of :

OVERDUE PERIOD

The foremost and most popular sign that a woman is pregnant is when her yearly period is missed. A woman's body begins to produce hormones during gestation that stop her ovulation and uterine filling from slipping. She accordingly experiences an interruption in her menstrual cycle, delaying her coming period till after giving birth. It's pivotal to flash back , however, that a woman isn't inescapably pregnant when her period is absent, an irregular period can also be affected by other effects like stress, heavy exercise, overeating, hormone imbalances, and a host of other issues.

Day(as well as pm. and a.m.)SICKNESS

Despite being known as" morning sickness," this pregnant symptom can strike day or night. before the first two weeks of gestation, nausea can strike. Nausea can vary in intensity and isn't endured by everyone. It's possible to feel queasy without throwing up. About half of pregnant women experience nausea and vomiting. While feeling queasy is normal during gestation, it can become dangerous if it causes you to get dehydrated.However, you may have hyperemesis gravidarum, If your severe nausea makes it delicate for you to swallow food or liquids. It's critical to get help from your healthcare guru if you are passing extreme nausea and dehumidification.

SORENESS

It's normal for your guts to grow sensitive to touch throughout gestation. You can equate the soreness you feel to the perceptivity you have right before your period, but it might be more severe. Likewise, you could notice that the regions girding your nipples,or areolas, begin to darken and enlarge. You may relax knowing that this soreness is only evanescent and will go down as your body gets used to the increased hormone situations. Also, you may find that your bra seems tighter than normal and that your guts have gotten bigger.

FATIGUE(sick FEELING)

During the early stages of gestation, feeling fatigued is a frequent circumstance for numerous people. The elevated progesterone situations are the cause of this sensation. Fatigue frequently goes down in the alternate trimester, which begins after the twelfth week of gestation, just as other early-stage symptoms. Still, for a considerable proportion of individuals, it constantly reappears in the third trimester.

REGULAR VISITS TO THE RESTROOM

Frequent passages to the loo , may be experienced. The need to urinate more frequently indeed before you realize you have missed a period. Your body has further blood than usual, which is why this happens. Your blood force increases and your feathers have to work harder to filter your blood and get rid of redundant waste when you are pregnant. Urine is the waste that your body also excretes. You'll thus find that you need to use the latrine more constantly .

CRAVINGS

Food can become highly complex during the early stages of pregnancy, leading to food cravings, constant hunger, and food allergies. Many people have recurring feelings of hunger or have cravings for particular foods. Some tastes and meals may make you quite happy at this time, but you might also find that you suddenly don't like things you used to like. Food aversions can develop during the whole pregnancy experience, leading to a disdain for formerly enjoyable foods.

HORMONAL CHANGES

You may have mood swings as your hormones continue to fluctuate. This can happen at any stage of pregnancy and is quite natural. However, it's imperative that you get help from your healthcare professional if you ever experience anxiety, depression, or suicidal thoughts.

The hormonal surge and increased blood volume during pregnancy are the causes of the changes you see in your skin. Some people might have a pregnant glow and a better complexion, while others might discover that their acne gets worse.

SQUEEZING

Additionally, you can get intermittent moderate cramps that resemble your menstrual cramps for a few days. It is important to contact your healthcare physician immediately if you have severe cramps that mostly affect one side of your body. This can be a sign of an ectopic pregnancy or another issue.

Accepting The Emotional Shifts And Taking The First Steps.

It's critical to put your physical and mental health first during pregnancy. Never hesitate to ask for help from your loved ones. Communicate frequently and honestly with your family, close friends, and spouse about your feelings. Inform them of your feelings. Talk about the things that stress you out the most and your greatest concerns. They'll be available to offer assistance. Don't forget to partake in enjoyable activities. Every day, set aside some time for yourself. Do what brings you joy, whether it's watching your favorite film or going for a leisurely stroll with a friend. Enjoy your favorite pastimes whenever you get the chance. Think about putting your worries and fears about becoming a parent in writing. It can be helpful to discuss these ideas with a trusted person. Determine which of your anxieties are unfounded, and make an effort to let them go.

It's critical to recognise the spectrum of feelings that pregnancy might bring. Emotions that may arise during this journey include joy, anxiety, and mood swings. These are all perfectly natural. It is imperative to identify any warning signals that can point to a more serious problem. It's critical to get expert assistance from medical doctors or mental health specialists if you have recurring symptoms of anxiety or despair. It's critical to provide a helpful environment. Be in the company of people who appreciate and comprehend the emotional transitions you are undergoing. This could occur at work or at home. You may create an environment that is encouraging and helpful by accepting these emotional changes and adopting the necessary safety measures. This will improve your pregnant experience and support your mental health.

Taking Care of the Developing Life Inside

Pregnancy-related care giving directly affects the brain development and long-term success of the fetus. To the best of your abilities, it is your duty to provide your infant with stimulation and a proper environment. Tiny brain cells that are formed 15 million times every hour before birth make up your baby's brain! Maintaining a healthy pregnancy is essential to your one chance to lay a solid foundation of healthy neurons for general growth. What then can you do to care for your fetus? Start by taking iron, calcium, and folic acid supplements together with a reasonable amount of high-quality protein. A growing body of research indicates how crucial your nutrition is to your baby's health both in the womb and while nursing. Make sure your diet is well-balanced and full of vitamins, minerals, and necessary fatty acids. Apart from the process of cell production, another important aspect of brain development is brain cell migration. The location and connections a brain cell forms with other pathways define its value, much like the neighborhood affects the value of your house. As was previously noted, throughout pregnancy, more than at any other moment in life, your baby's brain grows at an extraordinarily rapid rate. The brain's cells settle into their proper locations once they are produced.Recognise the value of routine prenatal care, which includes seeing your doctor, getting the tests you need, and keeping an eye on your developing child to guarantee a safe and good pregnancy. Keep track of your baby's developmental stages to gain a deeper knowledge of the incredible journey occurring inside of you, from the early construction of organs to the development of major bodily systems. Learn how to establish a strong emotional link with your unborn child through activities like talking, reading, and playing music. This bond can benefit both of you.Prioritize having enough rest and relaxation, getting enough sleep, and setting up a calm environment to assist both your emotional health and your baby's healthy development.

You may establish a healthy and conducive atmosphere for your baby's growth and well-being by using these loving practices throughout your pregnancy

CHAPTER THREE

Monitoring Developmental Milestones In Foetuses.

From the time of conception until labor, your baby develops and grows. It passes through several phases, starting as a blastocyst, developing into an embryo, and ultimately becoming a foetus. The cells that will make up your baby's heart will begin to flicker at the five-week mark, signifying that it is still forming. Your kid will start to develop normal sleep and wake cycles at 27 weeks, and by 39 weeks, their physical growth will be finished. This timeline can be used as a reference to gauge the size of your unborn child and monitor its growth throughout the whole gestation period.

Week One: The Initial Wonder.

Your ovaries release an egg, or ovum, during the first and second weeks of your menstrual cycle. Sometime during the third week, your partner's sperm fertilises this. After fertilisation, the fertilised egg separates into two about thirty hours later. It is referred to as a zygote at this point. The zygote slowly descends the fallopian tube towards the uterus as the cells continue to divide and multiply in quantity.

Week 2: Fertilisation Takes Place

This week started with your body releasing an egg. Within 12 to 24 hours, an egg becomes fertilised if a sperm enters it successfully. The fertilised egg begins splitting into several cells as it passes through the fallopian tube. It eventually makes its way into your uterus, where it starts to integrate into the lining of the uterus

Week 3: Implantation Takes Place

Now picture a small ball of cells growing quickly inside your uterus's lining of nourishment. The development of your baby starts with this amazing ball called a blastocyst. As it expands, it begins to emit hCG, a pregnancy hormone that tells your ovaries to stop releasing eggs.

Week 4: An embryo is present.

Best wishes! Now your bundle of cells is becoming an embryo. It will be approximately four weeks before your next period begins. At this point, which is usually when you would expect your next period, you may be able to get a positive result on a home pregnancy test. Your fetus is as small as a poppy seed at this point. It is important to protect them from anything that could impede their development at this time. Steer clear of dangerous chemicals, drugs, alcohol, and smoking. Additionally, take care not to overheat as elevated body temperatures have been associated with a higher risk of neural tube abnormalities, particularly in the early stages of pregnancy. Hot pools, steam rooms, and saunas are not recommended during pregnancy. The outer cells of your embryo are actively integrating into the lining of your uterus at this point. Through the openings this process makes in this layer, your blood can enter and supply your baby with the vital nutrients and oxygen it needs to grow. Your embryo is now surrounded by an amniotic sac that is filled with amniotic fluid. This sac protects your infant as they grow by acting as a cushion. What's more, the yolk sac in your tiny embryo generates cells that will eventually become the gastrointestinal tract, reproductive organs, and umbilical cord—all while providing temporary nutrition!

Week 5: Hooray! Some organs are starting to form deep inside your uterus.

A tiny embryo that looks more like a tadpole than a human is growing swiftly. The ectoderm, mesoderm, and endoderm that make up this embryo are the three layers that will eventually give rise to all of the organs and tissues.

The development of the brain from the top layer of the embryo, called the ectoderm, the neural tube forms the brain, spinal cord, and nerves of your unborn child. Together with tooth enamel, this layer is also responsible for the development of the skin, hair, nails, mammary and sweat glands.

The development of the heart and circulatory system are starting to take shape inside the mesoderm, the embryo's middle layer. The mesoderm also develops the muscles, bones, cartilage, and subcutaneous tissue of your infant.

The expansion of the stomach and lungs ,the lungs, intestines, and early urinary system will eventually develop from the third layer, called the endoderm. Additionally, it will develop vital organs including the pancreas, liver, and thyroid. In the meantime, your baby's primitive placenta and umbilical cord are already doing their part to nourish and oxygenate them.

WEEK 6: Incredible Development

The growing heart of your baby exhibits cardiac activity. In the next few weeks, you will be able to see the cells flickering if you get a vaginal ultrasound. At every prenatal visit starting around week 10 or 12, your healthcare practitioner will use a portable Doppler to check the heartbeat of your unborn child. You can see black patches where your baby's nose and eyes are forming. The appearance of ears is indicated by tiny indentations on the sides of the head. The growth of the tongue and vocal cords is starting inside the little mouth. Your baby's arms and legs begin as tiny paddles at first. They will elongate and eventually evolve into limbs. There's a little tail that emerges from the backbone but goes away in a few weeks.

Week 7: Further growth progress.

Your baby's eyes are starting to form this week and will soon be fully formed. The primary organs that enable your infant to see are the cornea, iris, pupil, lens, and retina. It's remarkable how these components come together in a matter of weeks. The digestive system of your infant is developing rather well. The oesophagus and stomach are beginning to take shape. Your baby's oesophagus, the tube that carries food from their mouth to their stomach, is starting to take shape. Not only that, but this week your baby's pancreas and liver are also still developing. These organs are vital to digestion and general well-being. The field of brain development is experiencing a significant upsurge. The neural tube has developed and closed on both ends. It will eventually become your baby's spinal column and brain. The forebrain, midbrain, and hindbrain are the three separate regions that make up the brain, which is located at the top of the neural tube. The fact that your baby's brain is developing quickly is really amazing. Throughout the whole pregnancy, it gains an amazing 250,000 cells every minute on average. The way the brain grows and gets ready for life outside the womb is just amazing.

Week 8: Movements are Observed!

Fantastic news Your child is beginning to move around! These initial motions resemble little twitches and stretches more. They are truly visible on an ultrasound and start to appear around week seven or eight. That being said, you won't be able to feel your baby move until between weeks 16 and 22. The movements aren't strong enough for you to detect them before then. Additionally, your baby is about to inhale for the first time! They have breathing tubes going from their throat to their growing lungs, which are the beginnings of their respiratory system. Furthermore, your baby's body is developing a sophisticated neurological network. Not only can these nerves communicate with one another, but they also link to muscles, tissues, and even organs such as the ears and eyes. It's an amazing process of development and progress!

Week 9: More and our baby tooth buds

Teeth buds are beginning to erupt.

There are 10 little tooth buds developing inside each gum. The twenty "baby teeth" that youngsters will eventually lose during their youth are these buds. These teeth will start to firmly affix to your baby's jaw in the approaching week. Your baby's brilliant white teeth will begin to show when they are between 4 and 7 months old. Though rare, some kids do in fact have teeth from birth.

The heart of your child is growing.

Your baby's heart has now developed into four fully formed chambers. A prenatal appointment may surprise you if you were expecting to hear the comforting, consistent "lub-dub" sound of a human heartbeat. Many parents say that their baby's heartbeat sounds like tremendous horse racing. This is because the heartbeat of your infant is around double that of your own.

It's the placenta that rules.

Your body is working hard to develop the placenta, a new organ, in addition to growing a new baby. The umbilical cord connects this organ to your uterus and your unborn child. Your placenta is now capable of performing the vital function of generating hormones that support the growth and development of your unborn child. It will resemble a giant pancake and measure around 9 inches in diameter and 1 inch thick by the conclusion of your pregnancy. While there isn't any scientific proof to support its benefits, some mothers may decide to eat their placenta after giving delivery.

Week 10: A Huge Progress

The primary parts of your baby's eyes, the cornea, iris, pupil, lens, and retina, are now fully grown. The eyelids covering your unborn child's eyes will stay closed until the 27th week of your pregnancy. Wonderful news! The teeth of your infant are beginning to firmly erupt from the jawbone. While a small percentage of newborns may only have one or two teeth, most begin to erupt between the ages of six and ten months. Your baby's brain is developing quickly at this time. Their forehead can consequently momentarily enlarge and sit higher on their head. They also have a brain that is roughly half the length of their body. Your infant is able to move their fingers and limbs thanks to synapses in their spinal cord.

Week 11: Our Extremely Small Fingers

Your baby's little fingers and toes have shed their webbing and become longer and more distinct.The essential organs of your unborn child are now all in their proper locations and are working as the first trimester draws to a close. The kidneys are generating urine, the pancreas is starting to produce insulin, and the liver is manufacturing red blood cells. Furthermore, the four chambered heart of your kid has fully developed and is already beating. The genitals of your kid will start to form at the conclusion of this week. The external sex organs, such as the clitoris and labia in girls and the penis and scrotum in boys, do not begin to distinguish until approximately 11 weeks of gestation

Week 12: Our Miniscule Foot

A few more weeks can pass before an ultrasound is able to clearly distinguish between boys and girls.Your child is starting to learn how to move their hands and feet this week. They can now curl their cute little toes and open and close their hands into little fists.The small fingers and toes of your baby are also beginning to grow nails. Like your newborn, these nails are little and fragile.The formation of the stomach and esophagus started in the seventh week of pregnancy. Your baby's intestines expanded quickly at the same time, even pushing against the umbilical cord. But don't panic, the intestines will eventually find their right location inside the baby's stomach as the abdominal wall closes.

Week 13: My baby can urinate

Your infant can go potty! They are now passing pee and ingesting amniotic fluid, replenishing the fluid every few hours.

Making a meconium

Your baby produces meconium in addition to consuming amniotic fluid. This is the first solid waste your baby passes; it gathers in the intestines and is black and sticky.

Growing bones and teeth

The lengthier bones and skull of your baby's skeleton are beginning to solidify. Their bones and teeth are getting harder.

Week 14: The muscles are starting to unite.

Brain impulses are working hard to tone the muscles in your baby's face. Such little characteristics have the ability to frown, squint, and grimace. Your infant can also make actions like gnawing and sucking.

The hair on your baby is beginning to grow. Far under their skin, hair follicles have started to proliferate. Soft, downy hair will begin to emerge from these follicles on their chin, upper lip, and eyebrows at about 20 weeks.

Your baby has flexible hands and feet and is highly active, even though you can't feel it yet. They're moving all the time, kicking and punching little things.What a remarkable rate of growth! You may have noticed that your baby's length measurement is significantly larger this week than it was previous week. But your baby hasn't really grown twice in the space of a week. The measurement at 14 weeks was different because it was taken from the head to the toe instead of the head to the bottom.

Week 15: Tasting Is Possible

Taste buds are developing in your kid and are connected to the brain by nerves as they grow. The taste buds of your kid will be fully formed by the time they are about 20 weeks old. Food releases chemicals into your system throughout pregnancy, and these compounds eventually make their way into the amniotic fluid. It's crucial to remember that your infant cannot taste the stuff you eat. Therefore, you don't have to be concerned about whether they will like the dinner you've chosen.

Your baby can move all of their joints and limbs, and their legs are now getting longer than their arms. Your energetic baby is always on the go, even though you might not notice it just now. Your baby's appearance gets increasingly human as they grow. They now have distinct fingers and toes, eyelids, eyebrows, eyelashes, nails, and hair. Your unborn child may be seen yawning, stretching, sucking its thumb, and displaying a variety of facial expressions if you could see inside your womb.

Week 16: We Have Sensitive Skin

Your baby's skin is extremely thin, nearly translucent. As your pregnancy goes on, it will get stronger and thicker, but it will stay translucent for a long time.

Scalp pattern development

Your baby's scalp's hair follicles are creating a pattern that will follow them for the rest of their lives. Their hair growth pattern is determined by this pattern. Your infant has all of their future hair follicles at birth because no new ones will grow after birth.

A beating heart

The heart of your child is beating rapidly, pumping about 25 quarts of blood per day. As your child develops and matures, this sum will keep going up.

Week 17: Growth and Bones

The fragile cartilage in your baby's bones is giving way to solid bone. It's critical to eat foods high in calcium if you want to protect both your own and your baby's bones. Consuming enough calcium lowers the risk of preeclampsia and hypertension in addition to supporting bone health.

Your baby's connection to the placenta, the umbilical cord, is becoming thicker and stronger. It will grow to a maximum length of nine inches and a maximum thickness of one inch at the conclusion of the pregnancy. Your baby's umbilical cord is vital for both eliminating waste and supplying them with nutrition. Your baby's skin layers will be fully completed in the upcoming week when sweat gland development gets underway.

Week 18: There is a clearer ultrasound picture.

Your child's visage,an ultrasound clearly shows the lips, nose, and ears of your kid. Not only do eyelids and eyebrows form, but also eyelashes, nails, and hair!

Lungs spreading apart,the tiniest tubes in your baby's lungs, called bronchioles, begin to form. We see the emergence of respiratory sacs at the end of these small tubes. These sacs will be packed with microscopic blood vessels by the time your baby is born, which will permit the exchange of carbon dioxide and oxygen.

Boy and girl portions

The uterus and fallopian tubes of a girl are developed and in situ at birth. In the event that your child is male, his penis is now visible.

Week 19: We're starting to develop an identity

The prints of fingers

Even if your baby is an identical twin, their patterns on their fingers and toes have grown into distinct, permanent fingerprints!

Your baby's perspective on the world, the senses in your infant are maturing quickly. Particular regions of their brain are being developed for taste, smell, hearing, sight, and feeling.

What makes Vernix Caseosa important : Your baby's skin is now developing vernix caseosa, a protective white layer. Vernix protects against hazardous bacteria, helps your baby's skin stay protected and moisturized, and supports the development of their digestive system and lungs.

Week 20: We Are Able to Produce Noise

You shouldn't be alarmed if your unborn child exhibits mild, repetitive jerking motions; these are known as baby hiccups in the womb. Most expectant mothers experience baby hiccups between weeks 16 and 22, frequently at the same time they experience other fetal movements.

Your infant can now taste things. They can send signals from many of their taste buds to their brains, and they are ingesting food particles that have entered the amniotic fluid through your bloodstream. Some research indicates that what you eat during pregnancy may affect your baby's later food preferences, though researchers are unsure if babies can actually taste these particles.

Week 21: Our Palettes

When your baby swallows your amniotic fluid, their functioning taste buds allow them to taste the stuff you eat.

You may have seen on an ultrasound that your baby can suck their thumb as their sucking reflex develops.

Even though your baby's skin is now transparent and wrinkled, they will eventually have smooth, lovely skin. Visible blood vessels are what give the appearance of redness.

When your baby becomes bigger, those first flutters will develop into full-fledged kicks and nudges that people may feel if they put their touch on your abdomen.

It is advised that you begin interviewing possible doulas as soon as you decide to hire one, as they are skilled labor and delivery aides who may offer assistance throughout the birth of your child. Because swimming is low-impact and soft on the body, it's a great workout for expecting mothers. It can also lessen the aches and discomfort associated with pregnancy. The weightless sensation of floating in the water is even more delightful as your tummy grows

Week 22: Mom, could you please see my hair on the ultrasound?

Your baby's little head is beginning to display hair. It may become thick and lustrous near the end of your pregnancy, even though it is thin now. In addition, your baby now has soft, fine body hair, on their forehead, shoulders, back, and ears in addition to eyebrows. Your baby can hear sounds that originate from inside your body, such as your heartbeat, breathing, and digestion. These will sound louder as their hearing improves. When your baby is a baby, he or she might sleep better with a sound machine that makes soft whooshing and thumping noises that are familiar to them. Your baby's skin is beginning to get covered with a layer of fat. Your baby's physique is still very slim for now, but you will love to kiss their plump rolls later.

Week 23: My Mother Sings to Me Now.

sounds from outside your body, like your voice or your partner's voice, can be heard by your baby. Research indicates that infants begin to identify and acquire a preference for their mother's voice even before they are born.

This is the beginning of the wave-like movements that assist your baby's digestive tract move food along. But at this point, it's merely practise for your baby's digestive system because there isn't any actual food to move.

Your belly may have begun to flutter gently, but now it might be feeling more strongly. Your baby's motions will eventually change from feeling like butterfly wings to mild jabs and kicks. You can begin observing your baby's movement patterns from 23 weeks. Do they become more energetic following a meal? Do they become slightly more active as you go to sleep?

Week 24: The Respiratory Sacs Are Forming

Your baby's lungs are growing and accumulating more respiratory sacs. By doing this, the surface area available for the exchange of carbon dioxide and oxygen is increased.

Your baby's body is gradually filling out in a balanced way, even though they look thin. They'll start gaining weight and getting more chubby soon. Their skin is still transparent and thin.

Your baby's face has little eyebrows that just began to grow a few weeks ago. They can now begin practising brow lifting and facial muscle movement.

Week 25: Becoming Adorable

Your baby's once-slim and elongated appearance will soon give way to a plump one. Their formerly wrinkled skin will eventually become smoother, increasingly giving them the appearance of a baby. If you could see your baby's hair, you would be able to distinguish its color and texture as it grows. The majority of your baby's day is spent sleeping, switching every 20 to 40 minutes between rapid eye movement (REM) and non-REM sleep.

Week 26: Quick expansion

At this point, your baby is beginning to breathe in and out small volumes of amniotic fluid, which is essential for lung development.

Your baby can hear you, and he or she may react by changing their respiration, heart rate, or pattern of movement. Your baby can startle at a loud sound, and you might feel them move. Furthermore, when babies hear music, their facial expressions change, as demonstrated by ultrasounds. The testicles of a boy you are expecting have begun to descend into his scrotum. It will take roughly two to three months to complete this journey.

Week 27: A Wonderful Turning Point

The wonderful milestone of your kid being able to open and close their eyes has arrived! Additionally, your baby may move in response to light. You may feel a flutter or wiggle if you shine a torch on your stomach.

Your unborn child is probably having hiccups in the womb if you notice any light, regular movements. These little bursts of discomfort are entirely typical and typically pass quickly. You can therefore take pleasure in this unusual feeling and not worry about anything.

Your baby's lungs are manufacturing a chemical known as surfactant in order to be ready for life outside the womb. This fluid aids in maintaining the alveoli—tiny air sacs—open in the lungs. This is crucial since it facilitates your baby's easy breathing after birth.

Week 28: Incredible Brain Development

Your baby's brain will grow remarkably during this trimester, tripling in weight. In particular, the cerebrum will expand, creating complex grooves that guarantee effective use of the available space inside the skull in addition to adding surface area.

Your baby's senses of touch, smell, and hearing are now completely formed and functional. Through these senses, they are able to perceive and react to stimuli.

Your baby's autonomic nervous system, which controls involuntary movements, starts to take on additional duties when they become 28 weeks old. It is currently essential for regulating your baby's body temperature and promoting regular breathing patterns, both of which are vital for the growth and fortification of their lungs.

Week 29: More robust bones

Your kid is taking in a lot of calcium as their bones become stronger. You should eat foods high in calcium, such as dairy products, cheese, yogurt, and enhanced orange juice. Your baby's skeleton is receiving about 250 milligrammes of calcium every day.

The myelin sheath that surrounds your unborn child's nerves is starting to mature during this trimester. This procedure will keep going long after your baby is delivered, protecting their nervous system. At this point, your baby's respiratory system is still developing. Their lungs are secreting a liquid known as surfactant, which facilitates the maintenance of their lungs' tiny air sacs open. Your baby's body will start making enough surfactant by the time they reach 35 weeks, which will enable them to breathe air when they are delivered.

Week 30: We are beginning to form our identity!

The color of your baby's skin is determined by the active production of melanin. The skin's level of lightness or darkness depends on the amount of melanin that cells produce. But the majority of melanin is produced after birth. Your baby's permanent skin tone takes about six months to fully mature. The hair on your baby's head may be longer than the hair on the rest of their body. Most of the lanugo, or fine hair, that began to grow on your baby's body a few months ago will fall out before they are born. Your infant can open their eyes wide, and they might be able to see faint shapes. By the time they are 31 weeks old, their pupils will have the ability to contract and dilate, enabling the eyes to adapt to varying light conditions.

Week 31: Finding the ideal dimensions

The required fat is beginning to accumulate beneath the skin of your baby, giving their body a rounder shape. Your unborn child will continue to gain weight as it gets closer to delivery for the duration of your pregnancy. Your baby can kick, stretch, and even flip over; in fact, their exuberant movements can be keeping you up at night. Rest easy; your baby is healthy and active based on all of this movement. Your baby's brain develops fully in the last trimester, during which time its brain weight triples. Furthermore, the cerebrum creates deep grooves that increase surface area without occupying additional space in the skull.

Week 32: Mineral Preservation Mineral storage

Your baby's body is actively storing vital minerals like iron, calcium, and phosphorus throughout this developmental stage. These minerals will be essential to the growth and development of your child. For the first six months of their life, or until they start eating solid meals, your baby will store iron in their body.

The lungs of your infant. Your baby's lungs will fully mature in the coming month. Nonetheless, your baby is using the amniotic fluid to practise breathing at this very moment. Their lungs get ready for the outside world thanks to this process.

Your infant's penis

A boy you are expecting has developed external genitalia and his testicles have started to descend towards the scrotum. However, if you are expecting a girl, all of her eggs for the duration of her life are already inside her uterus and ovaries.

Week 33: Mama, are you able to sense my movement?

Brain pliability

Your baby's skull has moveable, slightly overlapped bones because they are not cemented together. This facilitates the baby's easy transit into the birth canal, which is made up of your cervix, vagina, and vulva. Many kids are born with a pointed head because of the intense pressure placed on their skull during birth! The skull bones can enlarge during infancy and childhood as your baby's brain and other tissues grow since they do not fuse entirely until early adulthood.

The skin of your baby

Your child is becoming less wrinkled by the moment. As your child puts on weight in anticipation of delivery, their newborn skin is becoming softer and smoother instead of being as transparent and red.

Baby's motion

Your womb is getting tighter, which means your baby isn't flipping as much, but your range of motion should remain roughly the same. Your baby may kick you in new locations, like under your ribs on one side or the other, if they shift to a head-down position in preparation for delivery.

Week 34: Extremely Small Fingernails

Your baby's fingernails will have grown to the tips of their little fingertips by the time they are 34 weeks old. And at 38 weeks, just a few weeks from now, their toenails will grow to the tips of their little toes. So, keeping those baby nail clippers close at hand is a smart idea!

Your baby is developing a very cute baby chub as they grow bigger. They are getting even cuter as their arms and legs begin to fill out.

Your baby's senses are helping them to become more aware of their surroundings. They are now capable of reacting to touch, light, and sound. Additionally, their ears will be fully developed by next week, enabling them to hear even better.

Week 35: Movements of the Bowel

Aqueous Fluid

Your baby is encased in a quart-sized cushion of amniotic fluid at 35 weeks of pregnancy. Amniotic fluid production rises throughout pregnancy until about week 36, at which point it progressively falls until birth.

Gastrointestinal Movements and Urine

Your baby's kidneys have matured to this point and have been making urine since you were thirteen weeks pregnant. You might be surprised to learn that your baby urinates into the amniotic fluid! Moreover, your baby's first bowel movement is building up in their intestines.

Sleep Patterns

Your infant has developed distinct sleeping habits by now. These cycles may become apparent to you when your infant becomes less active while sleeping and more energetic when waking.

Week 36: Constructing Meconium

The lungs of your baby are ready to take on the outer world! Your newborn's lungs expand at its first breath, replacing any fluid left in the alveoli with air.

Your baby's bones are still far softer than an adult's, but the process of hardening them has already started. Some bones are made completely of pliable cartilage at birth, but as children grow, solid bone eventually replaces the cartilage. It's interesting to note that whereas adults only have 206 bones, babies have around 275 since some bones fuse together over time.The majority of your baby's downy hair (lanugo) and the waxy material (vernix caseosa) that covered their skin in the womb are falling off as they grow. Furthermore, these compounds are consumed by your baby together with other secretions, which causes the creation of meconium, a dark, tar-like combination that you will observe in their first bowel movements.

Week 37: Adorable Small Eyes

Your infant's looks

Your baby might have a lot of hair, anything from half an inch to an inch and a half, when they are born. Some babies, though, might only have extremely thin hair. It's crucial to remember that your baby's hair can differ in colour from yours. Furthermore, it is typical for their hair to fall out during the first six months and then regrow in a different texture and colour!

Your child's gaze

It's possible that your baby's eyes won't be noticeable immediately after birth. While some kids have their final eye color from birth, others may have slate-gray or dark blue eyes that, over the course of the first year, progressively change to blue, green, hazel, or brown.

Putting on weight

Your kid will be gaining weight in addition to growing. This extra fat is crucial because it keeps children warm after birth and smooths out their skin.

Week 38: Nearing Our Goal

Your infant's toenails and fingernails are fully grown. Your baby's fingernails may even reach the tips of their fingers, and their toe nails have grown all the way to their tips. Make sure you have those baby nail clippers ready in case your newborn has to have their nails trimmed soon after birth!

Looks fantastic

Your baby is ready for their first photo session: they have a wonderful layer of fat that makes their skin look smooth, they have lost most of their lanugo (with the possible exception of a small amount on their shoulders and upper arms), and they may even have more hair on their head.

Week 39: Out Soon!

Your baby continues to acquire more padding to help control their body temperature. Your child is most likely already 20 inches long and little over 7 pounds in weight. (Usually, boys weigh a little bit more than girls.)

When you grasp your baby's hand for the first time, you'll soon have the chance to witness how strong their grip has become! In addition, your kid can turn their head, has synchronised reflexes, and will be able to view your face when they are born. Infants are able to see things that are between six and ten inches distant.

Week 40: Gearing up to explore the world

It's hard to give a precise weight, although babies in the US typically weigh between 7 and 8 pounds. The average length is about twenty inches.

All babies have reddish-purple skin at birth, which eventually turns pinkish-red in a day or two. The crimson blood arteries that can be seen beneath their skin give them a pink hue. Over the course of a few days, their hands and feet may turn blue because their blood circulation is still developing. Parents with darker skin tones typically have paler skin at birth, which gradually becomes more pigmented. Your baby's skin will take on its permanent color around six months of age. Your baby's skull is made up of distinct bones joined by flexible tissue, unlike the skull of an adult. These soft spots on the top and rear of your newborn's head are called fontanels, and you will be able to feel them after birth.

Week 41: The Overdue Infant

Your baby has been in your womb for a considerable amount of time; they have reached the "late term" stage. They may therefore be larger than the typical baby. The majority of their vernix, the waxy, white coating that keeps their skin from drying out in the amniotic fluid, may also have fallen off. Your baby's size is amazing for 41 weeks now. Their projected weight and length are projected to be 8.35 pounds and 20.39 inches, respectively. But remember that these approximations could not quite fit your particular infant.

Dietary and Nutrition-Related Concerns During Pregnancy

There should be about 300 more calories consumed daily to ensure a healthy pregnancy. A well-balanced diet rich in protein, fruits, vegetables, and whole grains should provide these extra calories. It is best to restrict your diet of fats and sugars. It is possible to reduce pregnant symptoms like nausea and constipation by eating a healthy, balanced diet. During pregnancy, drinking enough of fluids is just as important as eating a healthy diet. It is advised to have multiple glasses of water each day in addition to liquids from soups and juices. It is advisable to speak with your midwife or healthcare professional about caffeine and artificial sweetener usage, as they may need to be limited. It is imperative to abstain from alcohol entirely when pregnant.

The Best Foods to Eat While Expecting

There are some foods that are very good for your health and the growth of your foetus:

Vitamin A and potassium are abundant in vegetables like carrots, sweet potatoes, pumpkin, cooked greens, tomatoes, and red sweet peppers.

Natural products like melon, honeydew, mangoes, prunes, bananas, apricots, oranges, and red or pink grapefruit are great wellsprings of potassium.

Dairy items like without fat or low-fat yoghourt, skim or 1% milk, and soy milk give calcium, potassium, and vitamin A and D.

Grains, particularly prepared to eat oats and cooked cereals, are significant for their iron and folic corrosive substance.

Proteins can be gotten from sources like beans and peas, nuts and seeds, lean meat, sheep and pork, as well as fish prefer salmon, trout, herring, sardines, and pollock.

Things Not to Eat

Certain foods should be avoided during pregnancy in order to protect your health and the health of your unborn child. The following foods are things you should not eat:

Refuse unpasteurized milk and any products derived from it. Soft cheeses such as feta, fresco, queso blanco, brie, Camembert or blue-veined cheeses fall under this category. It is advised to stay away from them unless they are labelled as "made with pasteurised milk."

Luncheon meats and hot dogs taste great, but be sure they're hot and blazing hot before you consume them. This guarantees the eradication of any potentially dangerous microorganisms.

During pregnancy, it's crucial to stay away from raw or undercooked meat, eggs, and seafood. That means putting an end to raw fish sushi. Sushi, however, can be enjoyed and is safe when prepared.

Finally, it is best to stay away from chilled smoked seafood and meat spreads like pâté. It is advisable to choose substitutes that are safe to eat while pregnant.

Recall that maintaining your health and the wellbeing of your unborn child depends on you making wise decisions during your pregnancy.

Guidelines for Managing Food Safety

These easy rules for safe food handling should be followed when handling and preparing food:

1. **Wash**: Make sure to give all raw vegetables a good rinse under running tap water before consuming, chopping, or cooking it. This aids in clearing the area of any possible dirt or bacteria.

2. **Clean:** It's important to wash your hands, knives, surfaces, and cutting boards after handling and preparing uncooked food. This lessens the possibility of dangerous bacteria spreading and cross-contamination.

3.**Cook:** Always make sure that beef, pork, or poultry is cooked through to a safe internal temperature. A food thermometer can be used to confirm that dangerous microorganisms have been eliminated.

4. **Chill:** All perishable food should be promptly refrigerated. This keeps it fresher longer and stops bacteria from growing there, which can lead to foodborne illnesses.

You can make sure that the food you handle and prepare is risk-free and safe to eat by adhering to these general food safety rules. Keep in mind that handling food properly is crucial to your health and the wellbeing of others you care about.

The Value Of Vitamin Folic Acid

It is strongly advised that women who are able to conceive take 400 micrograms (0.4 mg) of folic acid each day. A number of green leafy vegetables, berries, nuts, legumes, citrus fruits, fortified breakfast cereals, and some vitamin supplements include folic acid, an essential ingredient.

You can lower your risk of neural tube defects and birth problems that harm the brain and spinal cord by taking folic acid supplements. Different degrees of paralysis, incontinence, and possibly intellectual incapacity can result from these abnormalities.

Since most neural tube problems arise during the first 28 days following conception, this is the most important time to consume folic acid. But, as it could be challenging to diagnose pregnancy during this period, it is advised that you begin taking folic acid even before conception and continue doing so for the duration of your pregnancy. You should speak with your doctor or midwife to get the right amount of folic acid for your unique situation. For example, increased folic acid dosages may be necessary for women taking anti-epileptic medications in order to prevent neural tube abnormalities. Therefore, before trying to conceive, they should talk about this with their healthcare physician

Body Modifications and Well-Being

Pregnancy causes a woman's body to change in many ways. Many of these modifications go away after delivery. Certain symptoms are frequently brought on by these changes and are accepted as normal. But it's crucial to understand that some conditions, like gestational diabetes, can develop during pregnancy and that there are signs that could point to the illness's presence. In the event that any of the following signs appear while pregnant, you should see a doctor right away:

Abnormal or persistent headaches

Constant dizziness and vomiting

Noticing abnormalities in vision

Experiencing contractions

Having bleeding vaginally

Suffering an amniotic fluid leak, sometimes known as "the water breaking"

Edema in the hands or feet

Reduced output of urine

Any indications of a disease or infection

Tremors, which are trembling in one or both hands or feet

Fast heartbeat

Less movement of the developing embryo

If past pregnancies had early labour, it's critical to let the doctor know as soon as you observe any early labour symptoms.

Fatigue is a frequent symptom of pregnancy for many women, especially in the first 12 weeks and as the pregnancy comes to a conclusion. It is crucial that the lady prioritises getting more sleep than usual at this period.

Because progesterone is a hormone that is continuously created during pregnancy, the high amount of this hormone signals the body to breathe deeper and faster. In order to maintain a low amount of carbon dioxide, this hormone causes pregnant women to exhale more of it. Pregnant women may also breathe more quickly because their lungs' restricted ability to expand due to their growing uterus. The woman's chest circumference also somewhat increases as a result of this augmentation.

When exercising, almost all pregnant women feel a little dyspnea, especially in the later stages of the pregnancy. Exercise causes a greater rise in respiratory rate in pregnant women than in non-pregnant women.

Narrowed airways come from the lining of the airways receiving more blood due to increased pumping, which causes the lining to slightly bulge. As a result, the eustachian tubes, which connect the middle ear to the back of the nose, may periodically become blocked and the nose may seem congested. The woman's voice may sound slightly different as a result of these effects.

Digestive System

It's not uncommon to experience nausea and vomiting, especially in the mornings (sometimes referred to as morning sickness). High amounts of human chorionic gonadotropin and oestrogen, two hormones essential to sustaining a healthy pregnancy, are the cause of these symptoms.

Simple dietary adjustments and eating habits can go a long way towards reducing nausea and vomiting. These consist of:

Eating and drinking in moderation throughout the day in regular intervals.

Eating before experiencing acute hunger.

Choosing bland meals like pasta, rice, consommé, and bouillon.

Eating simple soda crackers and consuming fizzy drinks.

To alleviate morning sickness, keep some crackers by the bedside and eat a few before you wake up.

It's vital to remember that there aren't any particular drugs available right now to treat morning sickness. Hyperemesis gravidarum is the term for the condition that occurs when severe or prolonged nausea and vomiting cause dehydration, weight loss, or other issues. Antiemetic medication may be used to treat this disease in women who experience nausea, or they may even need to be hospitalized briefly in order to get intravenous fluids.

Other common symptoms include heartburn and belching, which may be brought on by a protracted stomach emptying and a relaxed lower esophageal sphincter muscle that permits stomach contents to flow backward into the oesophagus. The following actions can assist to relieve heartburn:

Eating less frequently.

Steer clear of bending or lying down for a few hours following a meal.

Avoiding alcohol, smoke, caffeine, aspirin, and other related drugs (salicylates).

Consuming liquid antacids; avoid those with sodium bicarbonate because of their elevated sodium concentration.

If You Get Heartburn At Night, These Steps Can Help You Feel Better:

Delay eating for a few hours before going to bed Pregnancy causes the stomach to produce less acid, which can heal pre-existing stomach ulcers and cause stomach ulcers to form less frequently.

Constipation is frequently brought on by the uterus's expanding pressure on the lower intestine and rectum as the pregnancy goes on. The elevated progesterone level aggravates this further by delaying the normal muscle contractions that move food through the colon. It is advised to follow a high-fiber diet, drink plenty of water, and exercise frequently to avoid constipation.

One typical problem that might result in haemorrhoids is pressure from the expanding uterus or constipation. Warm soaks, anaesthetic gel, and stool softeners can all be used to ease the pain that comes with haemorrhoids.

Pica, an extraordinary hunger for weird meals or nonfoods like starch or clay, can occur in some pregnant women. Furthermore, there could be an overabundance of saliva, particularly in people who also experience morning sickness. This symptom is harmless even though it could be upsetting.

It's interesting to note that gallstones seem to occur more frequently during pregnancy.

SKINNING

Melasma, sometimes referred to as the "mask of pregnancy," is a patchy, brownish pigment that can appear on the skin's cheeks and forehead. Furthermore, there's a chance that the skin around the nipples will darken. The development of a dark line, or linea nigra, down the middle of the abdomen is another typical alteration. These alterations result from a hormone produced by the placenta that activates melanocytes, the cells that produce melanin, the pigment that gives skin its dark brown colour.

Additionally, the abdomen may occasionally get pink stretch marks. This occurs when the adrenal hormone levels rise and the uterus grows quickly.

Expanded and thin-walled capillaries may become apparent in the lower legs.

Two rashes that can cause excruciating itching during pregnancy are pemphigoid (herpes) gestationis and pruritic urticarial papules and plaques of pregnancy, sometimes referred to as urticaria of pregnancy. Although it can occur at any time after the 24th week of pregnancy and occasionally even after delivery, the former usually manifests in the final two to three weeks of pregnancy. This condition's underlying cause is still unknown. Conversely, herpes gestationis, or pemphigoid, can appear immediately upon childbirth or after the completion of the 12th week of pregnancy. It is thought to be brought on by aberrant antibodies that assault the body's own tissues and set off an autoimmune response. Remember that not every pregnancy results in these changes.

HORNATES

Pregnancy affects practically all hormones in the body, mostly due to the hormones generated by the placenta. For instance, the placenta generates a hormone that stimulates the woman's thyroid gland to become more active and create bigger quantities of thyroid hormones. When the thyroid gland becomes more active, the lady may suffer a quicker heart rate, palpitations, increased perspiration, mood changes, and thyroid gland enlargement. However, the prevalence of hyperthyroidism, a disease in which the thyroid gland malfunctions and becomes overactive, is rare, involving less than 0.1% of pregnancies.

Early in pregnancy, oestrogen and progesterone levels grow because of the major hormone produced by the placenta, human chorionic gonadotropin, which continuously stimulates the ovaries to make them. By 9 to 10 weeks of pregnancy, the placenta itself starts releasing large levels of oestrogen and progesterone. These hormones serve a critical function in supporting the pregnancy.

The placenta also encourages the adrenal glands to create larger levels of aldosterone and cortisol, which regulate the excretion of fluids by the kidneys. This leads to increased fluid retention.

Hormonal changes during pregnancy alter how the body handles sugar. As the pregnancy advances, the body becomes less receptive to insulin compared to its usual functioning.

Consequently, the sugar level in the blood rises, requiring more insulin to manage it. If diabetes already exists, being pregnant may make it worse. Furthermore, diabetes that develops during pregnancy, known as gestational diabetes, may also occur.

MUSCLES AND JOINTS

A woman's body experiences changes in her muscles and joints during her pregnancy. Her pelvic bones become more pliable and loosely connected by cartilage and fibrous fibres. This is required to make room for the expanding uterus and to get ready for the baby's birth. As a result, the woman experiences certain modifications in her posture.

Backaches of various intensities are not uncommon in expectant mothers. This is a result of the spine curving more to counteract the weight of the growing uterus. It is best to avoid heavy lifting and to bend at the knees rather than the waist while picking up objects in order to reduce this discomfort. Keeping proper posture is also crucial.

CHAPTER FOUR

Managing Everyday Physical Discomfort.

Pregnancy causes a variety of physical changes, not merely weight increase and alterations in body composition. Your body's chemistry and functions change as well. For example, your body temperature may rise a little bit as your heart pumps harder. In addition, the body secretes more, hormones are impacted, and joints and ligaments become more flexible. Mood swings are typical, and they might be linked to both increased fatigue and hormonal changes. Anxiety about income, sexuality, marriage roles, body image, and approaching childbirth may also accompany these. Here are some tips to assist you manage the most typical pregnancy discomforts:

Vomiting and Nausea

Eat small, frequent meals to prevent the worsening of nausea caused by prolonged fasting. Try eating every one to two hours if you are always sick.

Stay clear of oily and high-fat foods because they are harder to digest.

Eat items high in dry starch, such as toast, cereal, and crackers, before waking up. After eating, it could be beneficial to remain in bed for about 20 minutes and get up gradually, since abrupt movements of the body might exacerbate nausea.

Sipping carbonated drinks and herbal teas with flavours like chamomile, spearmint, and peppermint may help.

Make sure your diet is full of items high in carbohydrates, such as rice, bread, fruit, and cereal. They provide you energy and are simple to digest.

Take prenatal vitamins as prescribed, but think about asking your doctor if you may wait a few weeks to take them if they irritate your stomach.

Distinct meals, such as milk or tea, elicit distinct reactions in women. Something that could calm one lady could agitate another. Nonetheless, compared to hot foods and beverages, most women can handle cold ones more easily.

Eating a high-protein snack before bed can help stabilise your blood sugar levels.

You should avoid drinking too much coffee because it can increase the secretion of acid, which exacerbates nausea.

It is advised to eat meals and beverages separately to facilitate digestion. It is advised to avoid drinking liquids for 20 to 30 minutes following a meal.

Bloating

In order to reduce constipation, you should improve your diet by including more foods high in fibre. These consist of nuts, dried fruits, whole grain goods, fruits, and raw veggies. Choose a cereal for breakfast that has at least five grams of fibre per serving. These dietary options support regular bowel motions and help to soften stool.

It's important to stay hydrated, so be sure to consume lots of liquids throughout the day. Beyond that, exercise, even something as basic as walking is a powerful way to ease constipation.Prunes, figs, or prune juice can be consumed for a mild and natural laxative effect. These fruits have inherent qualities that help to control bowel motions.

It's critical to refrain from using laxatives as a permanent fix. It is advised that you notify your healthcare physician if the previously suggested solutions fail to address the problem. Stool softeners that are safe to take while pregnant might be prescribed by them. It's also important to remember that iron supplements might make constipation worse. With the advice of your healthcare professional, the iron dosage can be changed if this starts to cause concern.

Tenderness In The Breast

During the first three months, breast tenderness is most apparent. The breasts get bigger and can have a lot of sensitivity. Extra comfort may be obtained by donning a supportive bra that fits well.

Common Urination

Urinating frequently is normal during pregnancy, particularly in the first and last trimesters. To lessen the frequency of urination, you do not, however, need to restrict your fluid intake. Unless you feel a burning sensation or experience pain while urinating, the increased frequency is considered normal and will gradually subside.

Lower Arms

Your calf or thigh is where cramps usually occur at night. One possible solution is to increase the amount of calcium you consume. You can consult your healthcare provider about taking a calcium supplement. When you're in bed, try stretching with your heels pointed instead of your toes. This simple action can provide relief from a cramp.

Heartburn

You should give smaller meals a try, but make sure to have them more often. It's recommended to keep away from foods that are heavily seasoned, rich, and greasy. After eating, it's crucial not to lie down totally flat. If you need to lie down, prop up your head and shoulders using cushions. Drinking carbonated beverages or milk can often provide relief from heartburn. However, it's crucial to understand that some antacids are not safe to use during pregnancy. Before using any over-the-counter antacid products, it's always a good idea to check with your healthcare professional.

Backache

Many pregnant women typically have pain in their lower back, which is a common occurrence. This discomfort comes owing to the shift in posture required to support the greater weight in the front. It is advisable to avoid standing in the same position for extended periods of time. One useful exercise that can assist in alleviating back pain and strengthening the power of the lower back muscles, which bear the brunt of the pressure, is known as the pelvic rock. Additionally, lifting the feet onto a stool while sitting might also bring relief.

Dizziness

An abrupt change in posture or a dip in blood sugar level can both cause dizziness or lightheadedness. Use these easy suggestions to avoid feeling this way:

1. When rising from a seated or sleeping position, take your time. To ensure that your body adjusts gradually, move slowly.

2. Continue to eat frequently and in a balanced manner. It's a good idea to always have snacks on hand if you are someone who has low blood sugar. Fruits and pleasant drinks are great options to help maintain stable blood sugar levels.

Shelling Of The Feet And Hands

It is very usual for the hands and feet to enlarge slightly in the final stages of pregnancy. Making sure you are consuming adequate fluids is always crucial. Try elevating your legs and feet as much as you can to improve circulation in them. This can be accomplished by bending your knees while raising your legs up against the wall while resting on a bed or the floor. This is a good way to empty your legs before putting on an elastic hose, if you're wearing them.

Including Safe Workout Programmes While Pregnant

The benefits of physical activity can extend to many facets of our wellbeing. It can elevate our spirits, help with posture, and support the growth of muscle mass, power, and stamina. It has also been discovered that consistent exercise can help improve the quality of one's sleep.

It has been demonstrated that including exercise in your routine during pregnancy has various advantages. It can lower the risk of preeclampsia, or elevated blood pressure during pregnancy, gestational diabetes, and the necessity for cesarean sections. Exercise during pregnancy can also help with healthy weight gain and ease some of the discomforts brought on by physical changes, like backaches, bloating, and constipation. All things considered, keeping up a regular exercise routine during pregnancy helps you stay physically fit, increases your energy, and prepares you to handle labor more skillfully.

In addition, exercising soon after giving birth helps hasten your recuperation and protect you against postpartum depression. You are proactively preserving your general well-being during this life-changing stage by continuing to be active.

Which Workout Ought to?

The most beneficial type of exercise is cardiovascular fitness. Pregnancy-safe exercises include jogging, yoga, Pilates, swimming, cycling, aerobics, and walking. Always be mindful of how your body feels, and make sure you're getting enough water to stay hydrated.

Try Kegel exercises if you'd want to perform additional exercises that strengthen your pelvic floor muscles, which support the bladder, small intestine, rectum, and uterus.

Is it Safe?

Yes, as long as a woman's doctor advises her otherwise, exercising is OK during pregnancy. If you exercise regularly before becoming pregnant, you can keep up the same level of intensity. Don't worry if you weren't active previously; you may still begin right now with easy workouts like stretching, riding, or walking.

Staying hydrated and avoiding intense heat are two ways to keep yourself safe when exercising. Additionally, it's critical to avoid contact sports and high-risk activities that involve falling, such gymnastics, water skiing, horseback riding, wrestling, hockey, basketball, soccer and diving. Exercises that require strong balance later in pregnancy or that need you to lie on your back should also be avoided after the first trimester of pregnancy.

The Sufficient Amount

A common recommendation from medical specialists is to progressively increase your aerobic exercise to at least 150 minutes per week. This can be accomplished by exercising for 30 minutes five days a week. If this sounds unachievable, though, don't let that stop you from leading an active lifestyle. Regardless of how hard you exercise, any kind of physical activity is good for you and your infant.

Take into Account These Guidelines Based on Your Level of Fitness:

Start off each day with simply five minutes of physical activity if you haven't been active in a while. Increase the time gradually to 10 minutes, 15 minutes, and so on, until you are getting at least 30 minutes in a day.

If you exercised regularly before becoming pregnant, you should be able to keep up your current level of intensity as long as your doctor gives the go-ahead and you feel comfortable doing so.

Which Are The Red Flags To Tell Me To Stop?

It is crucial that you stop exercising and contact your healthcare practitioner if you experience any of the following symptoms while exercising: vaginal bleeding, abdominal pain, painful contractions on a regular basis, or visible amniotic fluid leakage. Additionally, be sure to let your provider know if you get headaches, chest pain, extreme shortness of breath, or dizziness when exercising. Apart from that, well done on keeping your body in good shape for both you and your developing child.

Emotional well-being and mental health are important details During gestation, looking after your emotional and physical health is inversely as vital as looking after your physical health. You'll be better suitable to manage the difficulties of gestation and life with a new baby if your internal health is in order. Expectant parents may sometimes suffer from internal health issues like anxiety or depression during their gestation. Consult your doctor or midwife for guidance and backing if anxiety is snooping with your capability to serve or if you have been depressed for longer than two weeks. Maintaining your internal health throughout gestation can be achieved in part by eating a nutritional diet, getting regular exercise, getting acceptable sleep, and minimising stress.

Can Pregnancy Affect Well-Being And Internal Health?

The period leading up to parturition is both thrilling and delicate. It's quite normal to be alive about what the future holds while you are pregnant. Stress is normal, especially after you realise that this is a big shift that you aren't completely set for or suitable to handle. Likewise, gestation itself can be a stressful experience. You may have to manage physical and hormonal changes in addition to stress from antenatal.

You might be indeed more anxious if you've preliminarily endured a negative event, similar to a confinement. Gestation can increase the threat of getting an internal health problem because of these variables.

What Are The Possible Internal Health Conditions During Gestation?

Mental health issues can affect both couples both before and after the birth, during the" prenatal" and" postnatal" phases of gestation. Some people may develop internal health issues like anxiety, depression, and, less constantly, bipolar complaints during gestation. One in ten ladies and one in twenty males may have prenatal depression. Anxiety during gestation is also common, and people constantly feel depression and anxiety at the same time. The liability of passing anxiety and sadness during gestation can be raised by several variables. These can include having dealt with internal health issues in the history, feeling abandoned, having relationship issues, having been abused in the history or present, or having medicine or alcohol dependence . It's critical to keep in mind that anyone can suffer from an internal health illness, and doing so shouldn't be met with shame.

WHEN IS IT TIME TO HELP?

It's critical that all soon- to- be parents concentrate on their general good and internal heartiness. There can be both good and bad guests being pregnant. It's time to consult a healthcare provider if you have been experiencing depressive symptoms on a regular basis(similar to sadness or solicitude) for longer than two weeks. Likewise, it's critical to seek backing if your negative studies and passions are snooping with your capacity to operate typically. It's critical to get help if you observe symptoms of depression, similar to losing interest in conditioning or feeling helpless and unfit to manage. Passing constant anxiety or solicitude is another sign that you might bear .

In addition, you should surely get help if you start passing fear attacks or if you start engaging in compulsive or obsessive behaviours.

Managing My Mental Health During Pregnancy A Guide

It's critical to look after your internal health and heartiness during gestation. Consider what you can really handle before placing overdue pressure on yourself, and flashback to taking breaks when necessary.However, don't make significant life changes, similar as moving or changing employment, If it isn't absolutely needed. Speak with your doctor or health provider before beginning any fitness authority. Eat wholesome reflections on a regular basis to maintain your body in good condition. Be in the company of people who give you confidence and serenity. Try to refrain from using medicines or alcohol as a managing medium for stress; rather, find healthy managing strategies. Make connections with other awaiting parents to form a network.

CHAPTER FIVE

Controlling Anxiety Associated with Gestation   and Mood Oscillations.

It's common to   witness mood swings when pregnant. Along with eating well and getting enough sleep, talking with a health professional might be helpful.Pregnancy can be an emotional journey, but if you've ever wavered between perfect, unalloyed bliss and whole, maximum   anguish, you will understand. It's an stirring experience filled with happy highs and saddening lows. Indeed though not every expectant mama will go through similar abrupt emotional changes, those who do will need to learn how to roll with the punches and fight the appetite to knock someone out in the process. The good news is that mood swings are transitory .You'll be   suitable to be your calm tone at some point. We've some ideas and advice to help you figure out why you might be blowing hot or cold at any particular time in the meantime

Why Do Mood Fluctuations During Pregnancy Occur?

Mood swings can occur during pregnancy for a variety of causes, the main ones being hormones, lack of sleep, and persistent dread. Rest assured that there are legitimate physiological, psychological, and physiological causes for this erratic behaviour; you are not just being dramatic.

Do Mood Swings Indicate a Pending Pregnancy?

If you find yourself crying at a sentimental commercial one moment and furious over an empty ice cream carton the next, you may be experiencing pregnancy-related mood swings. A sudden shift in mood may be a sign of pregnancy early on. You can be caught off guard by your hormones suddenly exploding and your incapacity to regulate your emotions. If you suspect you are pregnant, this reaction may be exacerbated by anxiety and nerves.

Taking a pregnancy test is the best course of action if your emotions are erratic and you think you could be pregnant. Taking a questionnaire will provide you with a solid response in either direction, as many women experience comparable mood swings before the onset of their menstruation.

What Kind Of Mood Swings Occur During Pregnancy?

Mood swings during pregnancy might vary in appearance and sound. Both happy and depressing experiences could come your way. You can giggle uncontrollably at something ridiculous or become furious over the smallest of issues. You might have a hint of dread about all the potential "what ifs" of pregnancy and birth, or you might be resentful of your partner or non-pregnant relatives for being able to resume normal activities. Your emotions can be showing up as nesting behaviours if you are completely engrossed in baby preparations, such as building cribs, washing tiny onesies and childproofing cabinets and sharp furniture edges. Take care of your maternal instinct and relish this peaceful time of getting ready. Naturally, it's critical to differentiate postnatal depression from the typical emotional highs and lows of pregnancy. Despite tremendous progress in diagnosing and de-stigmatizing postpartum depression, a lot of women are ignorant that depression can also occur during pregnancy. For your own and your child's sake, you should speak with your doctor if you feel depressed, shocked, or hopeless all the time

While mood swings are a natural byproduct of carrying a tiny human inside of you, there are steps you can do to help you better control them if they're interfering with your daily activities at work, home, or anywhere in between:

Consume Healthfully

You are aware that hunger can cause unwelcome behaviour. With wholesome meals and satisfying snacks that fill you up and stimulate your mind, you can calm your inner rage and stifle your hunger. Having steady energy will support your composure.

Get Moving.

Exercise is a fantastic way to reduce stress and improve happiness. Consider engaging in some light, low-impact aerobic exercise, such as swimming or walking, if you find yourself feeling surprisingly depressed or irritable. Exercise outside gets bonus points because the fresh air will reenergize and rejuvenate you. Furthermore, the production of endorphins will promote happy and positive emotions.

Put Sleep First.

Getting enough Zzz's is crucial throughout pregnancy. Even while getting a good night's sleep might seem impossible in the first trimester, you can try to make the most of the sleep you do receive by adhering to a regular bedtime and wake-up time, as well as taking naps when needed. Do everything you can to encourage relaxation as labour approaches, even though you probably feel uncomfortable all over. Before going to bed, practise some breathing techniques and use pillows to prop yourself up whatever makes you feel somewhat comfortable (keep in mind, though, that side sleeping is optimal throughout the third trimester).

Speak With Your Family.

Make sure your loved ones and friends are aware of your feelings and the struggles you are facing. Tell them it's okay if you periodically lose your cool or have an unexpected reaction.By discussing this, you and your loved ones can prepare for more effective communication in the event that a problem arises. You can also think about making connections with other expectant mothers who are in the same situation as you. Participate in a neighbourhood group in your area or create your own online one using social media.

Be Gracious To Yourself.

Being pregnant is hard. It's more difficult when you're experiencing emotional instability. If you have a tantrum, overreact to anything, or are having a theatrical moment, don't be hard on yourself. Rather, practise self-compassion and gentleness, and remember that these temper tidal waves are passing. Everybody needs occasional emotional release.

Speaking With Your Partner

Maintaining open and honest lines of communication with your spouse is crucial when communicating.Many emotions, both positive and negative, might surface throughout pregnancy. You may be experiencing worry, excitement, or anxiety! Extreme emotions and mood swings can also be caused by hormonal changes in the body.

The Following Advice Can Help You And Your Spouse Communicate Well When You're Expecting:

Express your emotions and worries in an honest and transparent manner. Actively listen to your spouse and make an effort to grasp their viewpoint. Talk about your hopes and objectives for the upcoming pregnancy and beyond.

Prioritise your connection and make time for one another.

The Following Advice Can Help You Communicate With Your Family When You're Pregnant:

Establish limits and be explicit about what you require. Though you should be open to hearing what your family has to say, keep in mind that you are the one who knows what is best for you and your child in the end. Inform your loved ones about pregnancy and childbirth so they can comprehend your experience. Be compassionate and patient, yet stand by your decisions with firmness. Conversing with your pals,during your pregnancy, your friends, especially other mothers can be an amazing source of support. You can learn about other mummies' pregnancy experiences by associating with other mummies. It also allows you to know what to anticipate from the birth of the child.

Having effective communication is essential during a difficult period, like pregnancy. For a woman, becoming pregnant and giving birth is a transformative time in her life. Obtaining a lot of assistance and support will be crucial to making this stage successful.

Maintaining communication with your partner, family, and friends throughout your pregnancy is a great way to fortify your bonds and create a network of support.

Recall to be patient, truthful, and open; also, don't be embarrassed to ask for assistance when you need it. Pregnancy is something you can handle with confidence and elegance if you communicate well.

Settlements For Work And Delivery

There are numerous methods for getting your body ready for giving birth. You can try labor-assisting positions; practise perineal massage to lessen the risk of pregnancy-related perineal injuries; stay active to support your baby's posture; and acquire coping mechanisms for labor discomfort. Attending prenatal classes is beneficial as well. Breathing and self-help strategies are recommended for labor.

Position of Your Baby

The ideal posture for your unborn child to be in during the first trimester of pregnancy is with their head down and their back facing outward, towards your belly. The occipito-anterior position (oa) is this. Sometimes babies will lie head down with their backs to you. Working in this position may lead to a longer lifespan. The occipito-posterior posture (op) is this. The midwife Jean Sutton created a theory regarding the ideal placement of the foetus. She discovered that a mother's posture and movements during pregnancy can affect the baby's location inside the womb. Some moms employ these postures and exercises throughout the last few weeks of their pregnancy. They think labour will be much more joyful and the baby's position will alter as a result. The impact of these motions and positions on the baby's position within the womb is not supported by scientific data. The recommended treatments are secure and non-invasive.

Labor Hopscotch

Every maternity unit uses it as a visual help. Your physiotherapist or midwife might have it. The inventor of it was an Irish midwife. Find out about labor hopscotch from your midwife if you're in need of a visual aid. There are seven parts. Tilting your pelvis to improve the position of your baby is a common technique in these. Your baby may pass through your pelvis during labor. Exercises like lunges, squats, and sideways stair walking can cause your pelvis to tilt. There are names for each of the seven parts of labor hopscotch to aid in memory retention and relaxing techniques. Their name is: Stretching your pelvis to tilt it throughout pregnancy and during contractions is part of mobilizing yourself during pregnancy. To prevent your baby's head from sinking, use the toilet as a reminder to avoid and to help relax your pelvic floor muscles. Stool: this includes tilting your pelvis with a birthing stool. Water: this covers drinking enough of it while expecting as well as relaxing with water therapy. Mat: This refers to lying down on a yoga mat on all fours. Birthing ball: This technique entails tilting your pelvis by bending in a "figure of eight" while sitting or reclining on the birthing ball. Aromatherapy, massage, acupuncture, and homeopathy are examples of alternative pain management techniques (let the hospital personnel know if you use any of these). Entonox Tens devices also promote aerobic exercise.

When To Begin Working In Hopscotch

These positions can be started as early as week 20 of pregnancy. Verify with your obstetrician or midwife that you are able to begin these workouts.

These exercises and techniques can also be used during your contractions while you are in labor. They will facilitate your baby's easier passage through your delivery canal.

Positions and motions to employ when expecting from 34 weeks and beyond

ACT

If you spend a lot of time sitting up straight or on your hands and knees, try these poses while you watch television: place a wedge cushion in the car; sit on your side; swim with your belly down; kneel on a mat or pillow; sit on a birthing ball; or lean your body against a birthing ball so you are on all fours.

AVOID

A lap swimmer should not cross their legs.

When seated, avoid the "backstroke" and don't elevate your feet.

Pelvic Massage

The region between your vagina and your anus is called the perineum. This region may occasionally sustain harm during childbirth. Beginning at week 34 of pregnancy, massaging your perineum may help lower the chance of injury. After taking a bath or shower, when your perineum is softer, is an excellent time to try a perineal massage. To enhance massage comfort, try using an organic oil, like grapeseed oil. Avoid using synthetic or perfumed oils. Utilising a mirror during perineal massage may be beneficial.

The steps of massaging your perineum are as follows

Lie down and relax.

Press a thumb against the rear wall of your vagina. Put your index finger on your lower lip. Slightly compress in the direction of your rectum (back passage).

In your vagina, gently massage by making a 'U' shape with your thumb and forefinger.

There ought to be a stretching feeling. There shouldn't be any discomfort or Try to spend five minutes on this.

If you experienced a perineal tear during a prior pregnancy, let your midwife or physiotherapist know. Perineal massage should not be done if you have:vaginal infections, thrush, or genital herpes.

CHAPTER SIX

Understanding The Phases Of Labor

There are three primary phases of labor.. Your cervix is opening and your child is going down the birth waterway in the principal stage. The subsequent stage is the point at which

your baby is conceived and the third stage is the point at which the placenta is conveyed. Understanding the birth stages will assist you with understanding what is happening during your pregnancy.

THE MAIN STAGE: This stage the cervix mellow and opens, and this stage starts when the cervix starts to open. At the point when the cervix opens to around 10 centimeters, the main stage is finished. In the beginning phases of pregnancy, your cervix relaxes and turns out to be exceptionally flimsy. This can happen for hours, even days. You may not see anything by any stretch of the imagination during this beginning phase. You might encounter torment and uneasiness sooner or later, however there is no example and the constrictions are unpredictable.

In early labor, you might have a blood-stained bodily fluid release, lower back torment period-like torment that travels every which way free solid discharges, an unexpected spout or a sluggish hole of liquid from the vagina, when your waters break the 'waters' ought to be clear or somewhat pink. (a greenish or horrendous variety demonstrates a medical problem with the child, so you should see a specialist or call your clinic right away) a desire to upchuck (it is likewise normal to upchuck during pregnancy). Your body is planning for pregnancy in early labor. Things you can do at home: remain at home however long you can get customary snacks so you are renewing your energy holds; on the off chance that it's evening, attempt and rest by cleaning up or a shower; go to the latrine no less than one time per week and void your entrails (do a poo).At the finish of the primary phase of labor, you will end up being somewhat more fretful and depleted, and your aggravation will increment. The aggravation will be felt as waves, beginning little and ascending to a peak prior to falling ceaselessly once more. As you draw nearer to the subsequent stage, the time between each wave will be more limited. The time has come to go to the emergency clinic on the off chance that there are under three to five minutes between each wave.

At the point when to go to the Medical clinic It's not generally clear assuming that labor has begun. In the event that you're questionable or are concerned, call your primary care physician. Once in a while talking through your side effects will do the trick to quiet you down. On the other hand, you and the birthing specialist might choose now is the right time to see a maternity specialist during the conversation. The maternity specialist will ask you how and where you feel your contractions, how frequently they happen, and how lengthy they last. This will permit them to perceive how much your labor has advanced. On the off chance that you notice clear indications of labor, for example, your water releasing, sporadic compressions, or blood, it's really smart to call the medical clinic. It is for the most part better to remain at home in the event that you are not in business or on the other hand in the event that the labor isn't yet settled.

THE SECOND STAGE: This subsequent stage alludes to the period from when the cervix is completely expanded to when the child is conceived. In the subsequent stage, you might have: longer and more grounded constrictions, with a one to brief in the middle of between expanded tension. The need or want to prompt unsteady issues, queasiness and spewing, and consuming sensations in your vagina. In the subsequent stage, focus on your constrictions and in the middle between. attempt various positions - sitting, standing, or strolling in the event that you feel hot, a virus face washer can be extremely mitigating, a shower can be useful in quieting the aggravation, keep up your liquids and rest when you can.

LABOR AND BIRTH IN WATER: numerous emergency clinics today offer the capacity to labor in a shower. This will assist with unwinding and torment the board for some ladies. Ladies can likewise be saved in the shower for the birth in certain clinics. This will for the most part rely upon the accessibility of a certified maternity specialist or obstetrician who is guaranteed water birth and whether your pregnancy is working out in a good way. During the birthing system, the maternity specialist needs close contact with your child and should have the option to get you out of the shower in the event that there are any issues. Water birth is exceptionally protected assuming these essentials are met. Assuming it is viewed as safe for yourself as well as your child to labor and birth in water at the ladies' middle, you can decide to labor and birth in water.

PUSHING: When the desire to push shows up it very well may overpower. The pushing stage fluctuates for every lady and can keep going for as long as two hours, normally less on the off chance that you have had a child previously. Beside the desire to push, you are probably going to feel: pressure, and a compelling impulse to do a crap extending and consuming in your vagina. The child's head dropped down. Everything you can manage during this stage is to attempt to inhale profoundly, unwind and follow your body's inclination to push. Trust and stand by listening to your maternity specialist who will direct you.

THE THIRD STAGE This stage starts after your child is conceived and completes when the placenta has been conveyed. In the third stage you might have: more compressions to oust the placenta, a sensation of completion in your vagina. The birthing specialist will normally pull on the rope to convey the placenta however may request that you help by tenderly pushing. Recuperation starts during the initial 2-3 hours after conveyance. During this time, the uterus contracts to a great extent, pushing out what's left inside and restoring muscle tone. These constrictions are rushed by breastfeeding, which animates the development of oxytocin. During this time, you might insight: Quakes and chills, uneasiness from episiotomy, tears, or hemorrhoids ,Shortcoming and discombobulation, particularly while standing up,difficulty peeing because of enlarging in the genital area,when you can, you might clean up and afterward rest while recuperating from the pressure of labor. You can likewise begin breastfeeding on a case by case basis. Keeping skin-to-skin contact with the child is the most effective way to assist the child with figuring out how to breastfeed and keep them warm and quiet. Your accomplice can likewise utilize skin-to-skin contact to assist with keeping the child warm in the event that you don't feel like it. Your child will likewise be really focused on or observed during this time by a pediatrician. Making a birth plan and investigating conveyance choices. What is a birth plan? A birth plan is a composed outline of your inclinations for when you are in the process of giving birth and conceiving an offspring. It incorporates things like what position you need to conceive an offspring in, what relief from discomfort you like (assuming you really want it) and who you might want to accompany you at the birth. A birth plan can be an effective method for speaking with your pregnancy care suppliers about what means a lot to you before the birth. It gives them data about your inclinations during labor and what you might want to keep away from, where conceivable. Since you have no control over each part of labor and the birth, it is subsequently best to be adaptable in your preparation in the event that something doesn't go according to plan. Exploring labor and birth have the option to get clarification on pressing issues and will be presented to various birthing choices you might not have thought of. Ask the medical services experts about pregnancy care about their perspectives. Your choices may be restricted by your wellbeing, clinical history or where you live. Converse with different moms. You can begin by talking with loved ones however could likewise contact ladies who have conceived an offspring at the medical clinic or birth focus you are going to. You can get some information about how it went or what they would do another way sometime later. Converse with your accomplice or other birth friend. Talk about what sort of job they can accommodate you during the work. Find out about birth and your birthing choices. Go on the web and read about other ladies' encounters or perused books about work and birth. These sources will give you thoughts to talk about when your pregnancy is in danger.

A top notch and simple to-follow birth plan will permit your carers to see initially what is essential to you and what your inclinations are. A birth plan ought to be examined well ahead of conceiving an offspring.You may need individuals to accompany you during labor. This could incorporate your accomplice, guardians or sisters. You could have utilized a confidential birthing specialist or doula, or you could need your overall professional there in the event that you have utilized one under a 'shared care' plan during your pregnancy. You could likewise state whether you maintain that these individuals should remain the entire time or on the other hand assuming there are sure systems or stages in labor when you would favor them to leave the room. You can likewise list individuals who you don't need in the room. Climate Rundown a particular inclination you have for your birthing climate, for example, specific music playing, fragrance based treatment or diminished lighting (candles or stripped blazes are not permitted). Most clinics can oblige these sorts of solicitations however it merits actually taking a look from the start, especially in the event that something is vital to you. Labor comes with discomfort Note down the sorts of help with discomfort you need to utilize, which might include: rub TENS machine gas pethidine epidural. It is likewise valuable to record your favored request (for instance, you would like to attempt gas before an epidural).List any sorts of help with discomfort that you certainly need to keep away from. Keep in mind, this could change when you are in the process of giving birth. Positions for work and birth rundown any inclinations you have for birthing positions. These could remember lying for the bed, stooping, standing or hunching down. Notice in the event that you might want to utilize specific hardware, for example, a birthing stool, Swiss ball, mat or beanbag. Helped conveyance you should note down an inclination for forceps or ventouse (where a pull cup is connected to the child's head by a vacuum being made in the cup) in the event that you want assistance to convey your child. Conveyance of the placenta In your third phase of work, conveyance of the placenta, you might have an infusion to lessen the gamble of maternal draining or post pregnancy discharge. Record on paper on the off chance that you believe this should occur or on the other hand assuming you would incline toward a less overseen approach. Your child's umbilical cord gets on paper in the event that you would like somebody specifically (like your accomplice) to cut the umbilical line. You could likewise specify on the off chance that you would lean toward deferred line clasping. This is where the umbilical line isn't cinched or cut until after throbs have halted or until after the placenta is conveyed. Deferred rope clasping is an undeniably well known practice (many administrations presently do this regularly) in light of the fact that postponing the cinching of the line can mean your infant winds up with more blood volume than it would have assuming the string had been clipped right away. In the event that your child requires crisis treatment, postponed rope bracing won't be a choice. Techniques you might want to stay away from On the off chance that there are specific systems you might want to stay away from, if conceivable, posting them is significant. These could incorporate enlistment, counterfeit crack and utilization of forceps. Despite the fact that your inclination might be not to have specific methods, now and again they are medicinally shown for the prosperity of your child. Post pregnancy care check your maternity medical clinic or birthing focus' strategy for how your child will be really focused on following birth. Will the child be checked and tried first or will you have the valuable chance to bond with skin-to-skin contact straight away while the birthing assistant embraces tests? In certain nations, infants are regularly given an infusion of vitamin K upon entering the world; their most memorable vaccination for hepatitis B follows or occurs in the span of 24 hours of the birth. On the off chance that you don't believe your child should have these medicines you and your accomplice must comprehend the reason why these medicines are given and the dangers related with rejecting them.

Taking care of your child, be clear about whether you like to breastfeed or formula feed your child. In the event that you require a unique eating routine during your clinic stay or would like specifics when your child is conceived, have these nitty gritty in your plan. Discussing your arrangement with your health provider a long time before the birth implies you will have another person in the birthing suite who knows about your desires and can assist with conveying what you need upon the arrival of the birth. The main thing to recall about a birth plan is that births don't generally go as planned always! Startling complexities might emerge or you could alter your perspective once you are in the labor room. A few ladies are unyielding about declining all labor torment easing drugs however alter their perspective once they experience the aggravation. Adjusting your perspective is OK.You might have your heart set on a home birth yet your clinical history could mean it is simply unsafe. Clinical issues that arise during your work could mean you need to have a cesarean section or that your vaginal birth needs some assistance - like forceps. Be accessible to last-minute changes. Your prosperity and the strength of your child are the most critical .

Post pregnancy recovery and retouching you've been holding on for is finally here. Following a long time of supporting a child in your stomach and broadened timeframes of work, your little one is significant until the end of the world as of now.

Well done! You just did a marvelously beautiful thing. As of now comes the change from pregnancy to post pregnancy - and chances are you will feel depleted, sore and to some degree fretful. In any case, what unequivocally might you anytime at some point expect ensuing to consider an offspring?Your body and feelings will encounter a ton of changes in the long stretches of time following labor. Here are a portion of the vital things to anticipate following conceiving an offspring and during the post pregnancy recuperation process. Post pregnancy recuperation course of events How long is the post pregnancy time frame? Regardless of how you conveyed your child, the post pregnancy recuperation period is for the most part viewed as the initial month and a half after labor. This doesn't intend that at about a month and a half you'll mystically return to pre-child condition. All things being equal, this alludes to post pregnancy mending, which is the actual recuperating of your body after birth. What amount of time does it require to mend subsequent to conceiving an offspring? By the six-week point, your vagina, perineum or C-area cut ought to be recuperated, and your uterus ought to have returned to its generally expected size. All through those first weeks, you'll encounter a great deal of changes - from new degrees of sluggishness to chemical variances. Also, you'll likely keep on seeing changes in your body and feelings for a long time after a month and a half of recuperation. Your post pregnancy body: How your body will feel and change in the wake of conceiving an offspring. Post pregnancy hormone changes ,hormones are your body's messengers that advise your body how to follow through with something and when to do it. During pregnancy, your hormones changed to assist with supporting your developing child and set up your body for labor. Subsequent to conceiving an offspring, your hormones are on another mission to assist you with mending, bond with your child and breastfeed your child assuming you decide to. The main post pregnancy hormone changes your body will go through are: Estrogen and progesterone levels decline when your child and the placenta are conveyed. Oxytocin - known as the holding chemical - floods and adds to major areas of strength for the intuition you'll feel. Prolactin increments to flag milk creation. Draining and vaginal release As your uterus sheds that thick coating it kept up with during your pregnancy, you'll encounter some vaginal draining and release - which is known as lochia. Regardless of whether you had a cesarean (C-sections), you'll encounter draining and discharge.Lochia will begin as radiant red for a little while before steadily blurring to pink, and afterward light brown or light yellow. Draining and release will be the heaviest inside the initial few days in the wake of having your child, however will become lighter over the long haul. Regularly, lochia can last 4 a month and a half, with release persistently diminishing.How much draining is excessively? From the beginning, it might appear as though you're draining a great deal like having an extremely weighty period. This is absolutely ordinary, yet there are a couple of signs to look for. Assuming you're drenching through one cushion an hour for over two hours, call the attendant line or your consideration supplier immediately. Likewise, in the event that you keep on having horrendous releases or pass blood clumps for over about a month, call your consideration supplier. Expanded draining after your lochia begins to decrease can be a sign you're getting out of hand and need more rest. Seeing continuous clusters could mean your uterus is experiencing difficulty returning to its pre-pregnancy size. Regardless, it's in every case best to call. When could you at any point anticipate your most memorable post pregnancy period? A few elements can influence when you get your most memorable period in the wake of conceiving an offspring. One of the greatest variables is whether you've decided to breastfeed your child and if your breastmilk is their main food source. Ordinarily, the people who don't breastfeed may anticipate that their period should return sooner than the individuals who do ,Somewhere in the range of four weeks to 90 days subsequent to conceiving an offspring. For those that do breastfeed, some might get their period inside that equivalent time span - however many may not get their period until they've started to wean or quit breastfeeding completely. Vaginal and perineum irritation Both your vagina and your perineum (the region between your vagina and rectum) will feel exceptionally delicate and sore from the kind of labor. On the off chance that you conceived an offspring vaginally, it'll likely take you half a month to recuperate, particularly assuming that your perineum tore or you had an episiotomy. Assuming you toiled or pushed by any stretch of the imagination, however in the end conceived an offspring by C-section, almost certainly, you'll in any case be sore. In our "Post pregnancy basics" area underneath, we'll discuss how you might ease post pregnancy vaginal agony, and advance recuperating. After-birth torments (compressions) withdrawals after birth, additionally called after-birth torments, may be awkward on occasion yet not at all like what you might have encountered during work. All things considered, withdrawals after birth are flagging something great. After-birth withdrawals assist with decreasing uterine dying, and assist with contracting your uterus back to its standard thing, pre-child size. You might see after-birth torments the most in the event that you breastfeed..This is on the grounds that breastfeeding makes your body discharge oxytocin, a hormone that causes uterine withdrawals. Engorged breasts have been changing starting from the start of your pregnancy. What's more, around the third or fourth day in the wake of conceiving an offspring, you'll see the following large change as your breast will begin loading up with milk. Your breast might become engorged and feel firm, enlarged and sore. That underlying snugness and irritation will wear off regardless of whether you decide to breastfeed. Yet, assuming you decide to breastfeed, your breast will generally feel full prior to taking care of your baby .

Furthermore, you might encounter a greater amount of that delicate, weighty inclination assuming that your next breastfeeding is somewhat late. Sore or broken areolas blood stream to your areolas increments all through your pregnancy, so you've most likely seen some delicacy for a considerable length of time. In any case, the initial not many days in the wake of conceiving an offspring brings that blood stream to another level, making them especially delicate. What's more, normally, assuming you decide to breastfeed, that will have an effect, as well. As your child figures out how to appropriately hook on to your bosom, encountering a little aggravation at first is normal. However, when a child gets a decent lock, that ought to disappear. A little inconvenience as a child gets into a beat is ordinary, yet feeling constant torment all through your taking care of isn't. On the off chance that you find that you have breastfeeding issues, a lactation specialist can be a major assistance - and you can request one solidly in the medical clinic. Sore muscles You've recently completed the mother, everything being equal, so it's generally expected to feel some muscle irritation all through your body following birth. Furthermore, you might feel the eventual outcomes of your diligent effort for a couple of days. You can hope to feel particularly sore any place you hold a great deal of pressure during work, like in your arms, neck or jaw. Sluggishness, weakness is another totally ordinary post pregnancy side effect. Once more, your body has quite recently gone through (and is as yet going through) a great deal, so it's vital to get it as need might arise. Many consideration suppliers suggest dozing at whatever point your child does. You and your child's prosperity are the main things at the present time. Practicing good eating habits and remaining hydrated will likewise help you reestablish and keep up with your energy levels over the long run.

Night sweats many individuals experience post pregnancy night sweats because of evolving hormones. While they can be awkward, they are nothing to stress over. Simply ensure you're drinking sufficient water and attempt to remain cool. Night sweats ought to die down in two or three weeks. Lower stomach pain close to your entry point (in the event that you had a C-section) After a C-sections , you will feel discomfort and delicacy on and close to your cut, particularly for the initial not many long stretches of time as you recuperate.C-section recuperation timetable The post pregnancy recuperation process after a C-sections will in general be a digit longer than a vaginal birth. You'll probably remain in the medical clinic for an additional day, and you'll have specific limitations on twisting and lifting. You may likewise be recommended pain relief to take for one to two weeks after birth . Before you return home, you'll get point by point directions for how to really focus on your cut and advance recovery. Your entry point ought to be recuperated something like a month and a half subsequent to conceiving an offspring. Really focusing on your C-section cut while dealing with your entry point, it's essential to be just about as delicate as conceivable while keeping it perfect and dry.

This might mean, cleaning your cut on more than one occasion per day with a gentle cleanser. Either run cleanser and water over it in the shower, or delicately utilize a washcloth or shower wipe. Touching away overabundant water with a perfect towel, then, at that point, air drying the rest. Wearing dressing swathes to ingest waste and safeguard your garments, and changing the cloth day to day or on the other hand assuming it gets wet. How your temperament, disposition and feelings can change after labor. Having another child can bring a large number of feelings alongside it. Obviously, it will be wonderful and energizing, but on the other hand putting new tensions on you, your time and your energy is going. The following several progressions you can anticipate. You're probably going to encounter some blue eyes. After all the energy and magnificence of birth, it tends to be amazing and confounding to feel episodes of trouble, tension or peevishness unexpectedly. However, this isn't simply typical, it's extraordinarily normal.

Truth be told, around 80% of new mothers experience a scope of feelings or emotional episodes during their most memorable days with their child. Known as the blue eyes. The blue eyes may likewise give you sleep deprivation or cause you to feel overpowered on occasion. In any case, they typically disappear on their own in two weeks or less. During this time, being especially kind to yourself is significant. It can assist with conversing with your accomplice or friends and family about how you feel. Share how you're feeling so they can uphold you and assist you with traversing it. Assuming your blue eyes last over about fourteen days or your side effects become more serious, call your consideration supplier. You might be encountering postpartum anxiety. Your advantage in sex might diminish There are a few reasons you may not want to get physically involved with your accomplice subsequent to conceiving an offspring. You're drained and investing a ton of significant investment on being an incredible parent. Your body might in any case be recuperating or encountering hormonal movements. Discussing what you're encountering with your spouse or partner can assist them with better figuring out your sentiments. Likewise, knowing when sex is viewed as protected again is significant for setting the right assumptions for you as well as your accomplice. How long in the wake of conceiving an offspring might you at any point engage in sexual relations? Commonly, you can start having intercourse - on the off chance that you feel good and your health provider says it's OK .Close to about a month and a half subsequent to conceiving an offspring. Remember that hormonal changes can make your vagina feel dry and delicate, particularly assuming you're breastfeeding. Utilizing an individual oil will assist with facilitating uneasiness. Getting pregnant in the post pregnancy period additionally conceivable? Regardless of whether you're breastfeeding and haven't seen your period yet It's difficult to tell when ovulation will return subsequent to conceiving an offspring, so make certain to utilize insurance.

Your post pregnancy visit is an extraordinary opportunity to examine conception prevention choices. You might see changes in your relationship with your partner. You and your partner likely realize that your relationship will change with your child's appearance, however it might in any case come as a shock. It's entirely common. Your lives are both different now, and it will take some becoming accustomed to. Transparent correspondence will be your best instrument as you both change in accordance with your new coexistence as guardians. Post pregnancy basics: What you'll require available as you recuperate ,your health provider will ensure you have what you want to start the post pregnancy recovery process during your emergency clinic stay. (Furthermore, they might try and send you home with a couple of things.) However there are a few post pregnancy necessities you ought to have close by at home for when you get back from the medical clinic. Relief from discomfort drugs - Acetaminophen (Tylenol) or ibuprofen (Advil) might both assist at any point ease a throbbing painfulness. Your health provider might try and suggest switching back and forth between the two meds during the initial not many long periods of recuperation. Simply ensure you adhere to their directions and pose any inquiries you might have. In the event that you've had a C-section, your health provider might endorse a help with discomfort medicine for you to require during the principal two or three weeks post-conveyance. Post pregnancy midsection band - Stomach groups utilize light pressure to assist with facilitating a portion of the throbbing painfulness as you recuperate. Groups fold over your mid-region, from your hips up to your ribs. A few ladies find that wearing a band diminishes their back aggravation, upholds their pregnancy-extended center muscles and takes some of the pressure off their entry point assuming that they had a C-section. You might be given a post pregnancy midsection band at the medical clinic in the event that you have a C-section. Permeable maxi cushions - Tampons will be untouchable until you've completely recuperated, so you'll require agreeable yet retentive maxi cushions for the draining and release you'll insight. 100 percent cotton clothing - Cotton is breathable and can wick away dampness. Since you'll drain on and off for quite a long time - and all the more intensely from the get go - pick clothing you'll be good with discarding in the event that it becomes smudged. You can likewise track down dispensable cotton clothing, like what the medical clinic will accommodate you. (Tip: Request a couple of additional sets of dispensable underwear from the medical clinic. Many individuals view them as unimaginably agreeable, particularly the initial not many days in the wake of having a child.Ice packs in various forms will be an effective way to get relief from pain and inflammation. You can even get wearable ice pads for your perineal and vaginal areas. But the classic ice pack wrapped in a towel will still do wonders. Ice packs can also reduce discomfort from sore or engorged breasts.

As your vagina and perineum recover, use a peri bottle or spray bottle filled with warm water to promote healing and protect any stitches. The warm water is soothing and will enable you to gently rinse off your perineal area after you go to the bathroom. You'll receive a peri bottle in the hospital that you can take home.

A sitz bath, which is when you sit in warm, shallow water, can also be used both to soothe irritation and clean your perineum. You can take a sitz bath in your bathtub or buy a kit with a plastic bowl that fits onto your toilet.

Hazel pads are great for soothing postpartum hemorrhoids but they can also help ease perineal soreness. Lidocaine is a local anesthetic and is used as an ingredient in certain sprays. These sprays can give you fast, cooling relief from pain and irritation caused by postpartum hemorrhoids.

You may experience constipation in the weeks following birth. A stool softener can be a gentle way to help things move along smoothly, and put less strain on your vaginal and perineal areas especially if you've received stitches. Nursing bras for day and night – Nursing bras are designed to give you comfort and support without irritating sensitive areas. They also come with flaps that open to make it easy for your baby to feed without having to remove your bra. Even if you aren't breastfeeding, a snug, comfortable bra that provides firm support will do wonders. Wear bras that do not have an underwire. Lanolin and nipple creams – These special creams are a go-to treatment for sore, dry or cracked nipples. They can be applied any time you're feeling discomfort. And many creams are made with baby-safe ingredients, so that you don't have to wash them off before you breastfeed.

Health and Care Stores carry an organic, herbal salve that our lactation consultants recommend, along with other helpful breastfeeding products. Nursing pads – If you're breastfeeding, it's common to experience some milk leakage between feedings. Even if you're not breastfeeding,you might in any case release a little colostrum or milk from your breast right off the bra. Nursing cushions fit easily inside your bra to absorb holes and assist with forestalling a wet shirt. You can get reusable pads or disposables relying upon your inclination. Both should be changed over the course of the day. Warming cushion . To the extent that taking care of oneself devices go, the warming cushion is a work of art. Leaning against a wellspring of delicate, centered intensity can assist with various throbbing painfulness, from your lower back to your breast.

Your partner, loved ones can be great assets for you as you recuperate. You have a significant task to take care of, so be prepared to request and acknowledge assistance with errands and whatever else.

CHAPTER SEVEN

The Underlying Very Few Weeks After Labor

The significant length of time after your baby is born is considered as the post pregnancy period. After labor, your body will start to recover and go through many changes as it recovers. A piece of these movements happen the greater part a month. So rest whenever you can, demand help from friends and family, and eat well.

What Happens To Your Body During This Time?

Your body could feel sore and uncommonly depleted for quite a while. You could continue to have tightening influences, called afterpains, as the uterus returns to the customary size, having your first breastmilk In the underlying very few days after your child is conceived, your chests will convey yellow fluid called colostrum. This is concentrated food, so your youngster will not need a ton at each feed, yet they could have to deal with it routinely (maybe reliably). Your milk 'comes in' after close to 3 days and you'll see that your chests get much more full. How much milk you make will add or reduce depending upon your kid's necessities. It can require two or three days for your milk supply to match these necessities. As you start breastfeeding, your chests may to a great extent end up being unnecessarily full (engorged). This can make them feel hard and horrendous. It can help with dealing with: your youngster often,wear a well-fitting breastfeeding bra ,put warm woolen garments on your chests or wash up or shower and take some paracetamol or ibuprofen (these are safeguarded to take while you're breastfeeding).

If you will not breastfeed, take the necessary steps not to convey or 'discard' the milk in any way. This will extend your milk supply and disturb it. If let be, your milk supply will settle inside several days.

BREAST CARE

Your chests change an incredible arrangement during and after pregnancy, so it's crucial to check them reliably and have some familiarity with any weird changes. This is called 'chest care'. Chest care is critical considering the way that some chest changes might be a sign of chest sickness.

CHANNEL

Sudden or very profound blood hardship and signs of shock, similar to faintness, wooziness, then again expecting that your heart starts throbbing astoundingly speedy Channel or defilement

Driving Resulting to Having A Baby

Yet again there is no norm or genuine essential about when you can start driving resulting in imagining a posterity vaginally. Regardless, it is ideal to hang on until any medication is out of your structure, you're not in desolation and you feel perfect and sure before you get steering the ship. It justifies checking with your health provider if they have a condition about post natal concerns lately.

You shouldn't drive home from the clinical center after delivery.

How Do You Feel About Your Body After Birth?

It may not disturb a couple of women, yet rather others could have critical feelings about their postnatal bodies. You could feel strain to appear like you've never had a baby, especially if you have seen pictures of mums 'snapping back' through virtual diversion. Regardless, really for most women their bodies will change after a delivery. Doing a couple of sensitive exercises could assist you with feeling far improved and increase your conviction. If you had an immediate birth, you can start a sensitive movement when you feel like it. This could consolidate walking, fragile stretches, pelvic floor exercises or swimming.

It's for the most part brilliant to hang on until after your six-week post pregnancy check before you start any high-impact figure out, similar to heart animating activity or running. Anything that you do, endeavor to focus on how you feel right now, rather than what you resemble. Your prosperity and it is certainly more indispensable to really focus on your baby.

How Really Does Post Pregnancy Impact Your Sentiments?

Having a baby is empowering, yet it's not startling to feel depleted and centered. Your middle could change. You could feel that you don't have the open door or energy for various things or people. You may moreover feel hopeless. Banter with your essential doctor in case you feel hopeless for an overabundance of a portion of a month.

Your Baby's Mind

During your baby's underlying relatively few weeks, you will contribute most of your energy dealing with, diapering, and calming your baby. You could feel overwhelmed every so often. It is ordinary to consider whether you comprehend what you are doing, especially expecting that you are a first-time mama. Newborn child care gets less complex with every day. After a short time you will comprehend what each cry infers and have the choice to figure out what your baby endlessly needs.

Adjusting To Changes After Pregnancy

Many changes begin during pregnancy, more critical prerequisite for rest suggested less late nights and less blending. Most conversations had all through pregnancy seemed to focus in on the truth of been pregnant, so there was similarly no moving away from the individual and second-(or third-or fourth-) hand records of presence with a baby

The fretful nights, ravenous hankering goaded from breastfeeding, broken chests at a kid crying, the difficulties of going out, never anytime being on time again, challenges completing even the simplest of endeavors, frailty to finish a conversation (and all conversations being about our children), no greater quality time with your partner. Then, becoming a mother. The ability to comprehend the degree of progress that was required from a mother in my new position, being aware of the stack of lifestyle changes was absolutely helpful, yet it doesn't exactly position a woman to adjust to the reality that this is her life now.

Review Transience

No two minutes are truly something almost identical. Life is consistently created. This is unprecedented data . Fundamentally, your baby will grow up and you could attempt to miss a part of the troubles; the challenges faced are continually joined by one of a kind few minutes.

Practice Affirmation

We will regularly fight with unfortunate change. Getting through is made by our affinity to grip pleasure and push away distress. By fighting with conditions past our arrival we hold ourselves back from pushing ahead, consequently remaining trapped in a subsequent that has recently happened and this can't be changed. Change to change takes time, so when you notice you are fighting ask yourself, "Am I combating change or enduring it?" what's more "Might a qualification at any point push toward simplify my life right now?"Teach others in regards to your challenges

You are never alone in what you are experiencing as a parent. A sensation of affiliation and a vibe of being seen are major when we are defying any kind of challenge. License yourself to open up to buddies, various gatekeepers, or your associate when you are combating change. While doing in that capacity, pick your support adroitly; someone has an amazing open door and determination to tune in and who can give you the fundamental support you need.

Outfit Your Inward Strength

Life is stacked with challenges. Stop briefly to think about past trouble; see what components aided (or upset) your adjusting, what you learned about yourself and how you grew actually. Each challenge you experience as a parent, when defied with a significant (yet bothersome) lifestyle change, is an opportunity for mindfulness. Investigate various roads in regards to pushing toward change unexpectedly. By allowing yourself to consider the necessity for change to be an opportunity to learn and foster you are supporting your adaptability.

Embracing Being A Parent

Embracing being a parent infers embracing obstructions. Embracing life as a parent infers embracing the planning up of our children and the obligation expected to accomplish that. Embracing being a parent infers sorting out some way to make a dinner menu so you're not stressing the whole house essentially in light of the fact that it's an endeavor you could manage without. Embracing life as a parent is communicating yes to the youngster who demands that you play with them, regardless, when your arrangement for the day is a mile long and playing Candyland is close to torture.

CHAPTER EIGHT

Bonding with the Baby.

Bonding happens when you and your child begin to feel significant solid areas for each other. You could feel unbelievable love and fulfillment when you look at your kid. You could feel particularly protective of your kid. This first relationship with you prepares newborn children to have a strong feeling that everything is safe and secure and extraordinary about themselves with others. They sort out some way to believe you since they understand you are zeroing in on them and managing them. Newborn children that have strong bonds with their people will undoubtedly trust others and have extraordinary associations as adults.

Bonding is a Cycle

Bonding is a Cycle that has been extended. You and your baby could bond inside two or three minutes, in excess of several days, or a portion of a month. Holding could take additional time accepting that your baby required raised clinical thought after entering the world, then again expecting that you embraced your baby. Understand that you can bond with your embraced baby as well as natural gatekeepers bond with their children. Simply unwind or feel remorseful in case it requires more speculation than you expected to shape a close by bond with your kid. This doesn't infer that you are a horrendous parent. However long you are managing your baby's basic necessities.

Ways of Bonding with your baby

Ways of holding with your baby has been expanded.if the birthing framework did easily, your youngster may be very prepared after entering the world. Find a time to hold and look at your kid. This is an unimaginable chance to bond. Other holding minutes can happen when you: Breastfeed. Accepting that you chose to breastfeed, your baby will become joined to your smell and contact during feedings. Bottle-feed. During bottle feedings, your youngster can get more to know your smell and contact, also. Hold your kid, especially skin to skin when you can. Look at your youngster straightforwardly without flinching. Answer your baby when they cry. Certain people worry about crying . However, you won't attend to your baby with an abundance of thought. Play with your child. Talk, read, and sing to your kid. This helps them with ending up being generally acquainted with your voice. Recognizing help from Others has been broadened. While you bring your baby home, your obligation is to manage your kid and bond. This is more direct if you have help at home. You could end up being incredibly exhausted from all of the new commitments that go with having another kid. Allow friends and family to take on routine undertakings like apparel, looking for food, and cooking.

Adjusting to the Solicitations of New Life as a Parent

Getting to know this new individual, and their inclinations and character, can be challenging. That is whether or not you're really feeling joy and joy at your youngster's appearance. Sometimes, the enthusiastic thought of commitment, and the sheer drudgery of housework, prevents you from loosening up and participating in your youth. Things will begin to die down into a model and routine once your youngster is between six weeks and two months old. Regardless, if you're finding it trying to adjust during these underlying very few weeks, the following are a couple of contemplations.

Stretch your legs

While truly zeroing in on a baby, occasionally can feel terribly extensive, so have a go at isolating them. One way is to go for a short stroll, whatever the environment, reliably, to thwart fretfulness. If your baby is crying, you could take them for a walk around their pushchair to help with settling off to rest. A distinction in view, as well as outside air and fragile action, will lift your outlook and your youngster's, too. Walking will similarly help you with blending. You'll probably start to see faces, and it's amazing the quantity of people that start conversations when you have a baby with you.

Eat well

Anyway it's tempting to grab the nearest sweet chomp while you're feeling exhausted, eating unequivocally will help you with feeling significantly better. It will help you with recovering from the birth and keep your energy levels all balanced out. Pick basic goodies and blowouts, as you probably won't have the energy to cook. Incredible choices are a pre-arranged potato with fish or beans, or a sandwich made with wholemeal bread and a sound filling, similar to hummus and salad. Eat food sources which release energy bit by bit, furthermore called low GI food assortments, for instance, wholegrains and results of the dirt. Moreover, protein as meat, fish, beans, eggs, cheddar, nuts or seeds, should similarly be associated with your standard food choices. This is critical whether you are breastfeeding or recipe dealing with.

Act normally

Make an effort not to be excessively unforgiving with yourself in case the apparel isn't done or the dishwasher hasn't been unloaded. Contributing energy with your kid is the most compelling thing. In case you have parts to do, form a once-over and cross every task off when it's done. Pull out all the stops. That way you can continuously send and consider what you've done, whether or not it's simply anything from your summary. This is clearly better than effective financial planning energy struggling with what really ought to be done. Settle for less in the early weeks to keep the strain off. Endeavor to review that your baby doesn't mind one way or the other on the off chance that the reusing is piling up, then again expecting that there's a dash of buildup on the rack.

Find comparable association

You could feel miserable and cut-off from your past way of life. Your baby's dad could miss his past way of life also, but there are ways to deal with staying aware of family relationships.

Staying in touch with other new mums you could have met through antenatal classes can be a huge way to deal with blending. You can share experiences and your baby will benefit from other associations, also. Likewise, if you haven't yet settled your association, there are loads of approaches to meeting new mums.

If you don't have even the remotest clue about a few other unseasoned guardians in your area or a post pregnancy bundle curiously can torment. Notwithstanding, most mums benefit a ton from these. You could think you'll be the only one turning up there with milk stains down your front and very strong sacks under your eyes. You could imagine that each and every other individual will hush up, control, and regulate infinitely better than you are. Be that as it may, you'll run over watchmen who feel something basically the same, while conceivably not more unfortunate, than you right now. Sharing and exchanging experiences of being a parent can really help.

Put down a specific moment to the side for yourself

Whether or not you can't rest when your baby naps, you really ought to repay yourself with a genuine break, paying little heed to how short it is. Have a rest from diligent everyday practice and help you. Whether it's having a shower, painting your nails, scrutinizing a book or calling a buddy, in case it energizes you, get it going. If you're incredibly depleted at this point and can't rest, have a go at shutting your eyes and loosening up for 10 minutes. Rest when you can and require consistently as it comes. Focus on our loosening up sound or endeavor some yoga loosening up, or any loosening up strategies you could have learnt at antenatal classes.

When will my baby sink into a day to day practice?

Exactly when people ask whether your baby has settled right now, you could think it a pariah thought, as infants and timetables don't regularly go together.

Luckily things will get more clear as you get to know your kid and track down what her various inclinations, and how she ought to be truly centered around. After a month and a half, you kid could begin to spread out resting and dealing with plans, in all likelihood without you regardless, it's working on a mission to comprehend. In any case, if your youngster hasn't spread out an ordinary this early, essentially unwind. A couple of newborn children need extra time and help than others. When a routine is spread out, you'll find it more straightforward to expect the day ahead, such as arranging visits to the office or coming to standard parent and youngster get-togethers. That is the place where you're likely going to feel obviously more in charge. Indeed, even though life changed everlastingly the subsequent you became a parent, the weights of the essential weeks don't persevere through all through youth. So in case your kid hasn't settled as of now, have certainty she will after a short time.

Dealing with oneself For New Moms

As moms, we regularly set ourselves last, ensuring first that everyone (and the wide range of various things) is managed before we consider looking out for our own prerequisites. We put on a bright face and tell the world, "I have this" - regardless, when we feel like we're missing the mark. We get a great deal of ideas to put ourselves first: you can't pour from an empty cup, put on your breathing gadget first, etc. Unnecessarily relatively few of us recognize this direction, and, shockingly, less of us create an open door to zero in on ourselves, as a matter of fact. It's not just alright to manage yourself; it's a need - especially when you're pregnant and post pregnancy.

Here Are Precisely Several Hints

1.Assemble your town.

After the ruckus of the movement and everyone clamoring to meet your youngster, requiring quiet time all together with your family is typical. At the point when you've placed in several days (or weeks) getting to know the unpredictable subtleties of life as a parent, contact your partners, family, colleagues, or neighbors. Most of your loved ones will cheerfully give their time or resources for two or three baby nestles. Give your folks access regulation or dearest friends bring dinner one day in seven days. Demand that neighbors help with managing the grass or digging instruments in the garage. Call an ally to get two or three things from the store for you, run a pile of dress, or take your canine for a walk. If it's in your spending plan, enlist a post pregnancy doula to assist with childcare and help you with having positive assumptions regarding breastfeeding.

2.Track down your space

We contribute such a great deal of energy setting up the nursery we disregard to remove space for ourselves. Create an agreeable specialty in your home where you can relax. Spaces with plants and standard light are perfect for loosening up, very much like the letting hints free from a smokestack, wellspring, bird feeder, or fish tank. A one of a kind seat or floor covering can help with describing a sensation of "place.

3.Reclaim your Day

License yourself a valuable chance to play. While it might be tempting to use when your baby's resting to find a good pace with work or tasks, you can similarly take two or three those minutes to scrutinize, work in the nursery, play with pets, get ready, sew, paint, dance, sing, or whatever else you appreciate. What's more, don't underestimate the recovering power of a shower or shower. Having a companion or relative watch your baby for 30 minutes so you can retain the tub or wash up fundamentally influences your ability to loosen up. Add plants, fragrant mending, relaxing nature sounds, or candles to make a spa-like climate in your bathroom. Yet again occasionally a quick shower is all you truly need to feel human. Moreover, if no one's open to watch your kid, keep a bouncer in the bathroom so you can sneak in to wash your hair.

4. Get away from the house and take an endeavor.

Plan time with your allies to get away from the house: get some coffee, get a pedicure, eat, walk around the recreation area, or see a film. Make your time together a custom so it doesn't drop off the radar. Assuming your baby values riding in the vehicle or carriage, use that chance to research. Head off on an excursion; find a spot you've never been or reliably expected to see. On the other hand, branch out alone. Leave your kid home with family and require several hours to go to someplace you really want to go. Cut out a potential open door to do things you loved before kid.

5. Seek after an energy with your association.

Our lives are so involved and full it's quite easy to fail to focus on our associations. Strong Associations take work, time, and objectives. Scorn can race to the surface expecting you and your association to quit conveying, especially about the particular qualities you love around each other. Maybe you love cooking, so you expect to make dinner together one time each week; if you value practice you can get comfortable with another game together. Regardless, zeroing in on a without screen night to focus in on each other can make a colossal difference.

6. Carve out some time for reflection.

Find several minutes consistently for reflection and examination. You can do this before your baby gets up, during the underlying several snapshots of naptime, or constantly end. Pondering your regular fights and wins enables you to fill in astonishing ways.

7. Outfit yourself with data.

A portion of the time you can feel so slowed down by the tension of figuring how to parent "at work" that chance to relax doesn't help. What you need then isn't actually "a break." You could require counsel.

8. Be minding to Yourself

Sustaining is a tough spot. It's not startling to feel hopeless, skeptical, or angry once in a while, so don't be challenging yourself about those opinions. Revolve around the things you have some command over and celebrate little victories. Review that a super second doesn't make an extraordinary day or an extreme life.

Your baby may not really need embraces and nestles, and at some point they'll make a beeline for rest without whimpering. Nothing perseveres forever and always.

CHAPTER NINE

Mental Change: Obliging Pre-baby And Post-baby Character

Experiencing a personal crisis of sorts during the start of parenthood is ordinary. There might be minutes when you completely search in the mirror and wonder, who is this person? The woman you see is someone whose entire life by and by seems to pivot around feedings, diaper changes, and rest plans. While the unlimited love you feel for your kid is unequaled, it's alright to botch the open door and promptness you had already. Mourning your past way of life doesn't make you a horrible mother; it makes you human.

The Meaning of Resistance And Self-Assessment

Being a parent is definitely not a run; it's a significant distance race. The promising and less promising times come in waves, and comparably as you suspect you have everything figured out, another test — like getting teeth or infant kid reflux will come to prompt you that this journey is a perpetual assumption to learn and adjust. No one has all of the reactions, not even that supermom stalwart who appears to have the best life on Instagram. Give yourself a little space to breathe. It's alright to demand help, and it's okay to surrender that you don't have everything in line. To be sure no one does.

Embracing Your New Normal

Your new normal will be massively not equivalent to what you've known, and that is totally fine. Honestly, it's more than alright — it's your uncommon and individual outing, suggested solely for yourself as well as your friends and family. This new fact of the matter is a blend of your previous existence experiences and the wonderful complexities of being a parent. A constantly changing scene will continue to form as you form into your occupation as a mother. Enduring this can be freeing and will allow you to change all the more perfectly to the storm of shifts that come your course.

In this new period of life, balance doesn't mean doing everything flawlessly; it infers doing everything possible with what you have, and pardoning yourself for the rest. It's a layered, nuanced process that takes time, diligence, and a lot of confidence. Additionally, review that, you're following in some admirable people's footsteps in this — consistently, new moms especially like you are investigating their extraordinary labyrinths, tracking down alarming fortunes at every redirection.

Setting Sensible Presumptions

Life as a parent, particularly for new moms, much of the time comes encased by a radiant packaging of social presumptions and deliberate norms. There's an overwhelming strain to get it 'on the cash,' from supporting your kid to keeping up working and keeping an optimal home. However, we ought to uncloak a couple of legends and settle any falsehood.

Typical Dreams and Disarrays About Being a Parent

From kids consistently conveying couples closer to extraordinary moms don't need support, misinformed decisions thrive. Confining the driving forward through dreams from the fascinating genuine elements of parenthood is huge. Busting these legends eases your mental weight as well as accounts for a more genuine supporting experience.

Avoiding the Connection Trap

It's essentially a commonplace to look at others and can't resist the urge to contemplate how they're doing everything. Especially during a period of online diversion, where genuinely faultless families have all the earmarks of being the norm. Nonetheless, recall, assessment is the cheat of enjoyment. Behind each isolated photo, as drained and overwhelmed there's a mother's as you might feel now.

Utilizing Time Gainfully: The Dream Of Performing Different Assignments

The art of doing everything with the exception of accomplishing nothing totally. Studies recommend that performing different assignments every now and again achieves lower quality outcomes. Taking everything into account, it revolves around separated attention. Center around your tasks and proposition each one you're bound together thought, regardless of how brief that might be. Your work, your baby, and specifically, you, will benefit from this more cautious technique

The Impact Of Being a Parent On Opinion

The presence of one more relative most certainly moves the components of a relationship. Nights out and unconstrained departures might be sparse, and conversation could perilously float into a ceaseless circle of youngster talk. However, it's noteworthy that a strong association shapes the underpinning of an euphoric family.

Meaning Of Open Communication And Reliable Consolation

You and your association are co-pilots on this trip, and clear correspondence is your best course gadget. Track down an open door to straightforwardly inspect your sensations of fear, suspicions, and everyday successes. Lean on each other and give each other space when necessary. Near and dear openness will help you with getting through even the most anxious storms.

Arranged Us Time and Why It's Fundamental

In the disarray of new life as a parent, opinion could have all the earmarks of being a luxury. However, think of it as significant help. Especially like you plan feedings and rests for the baby, pencil in some uninterrupted time with your partner. It needn't bother to be a superb evening out on the town — a fundamental cup of coffee together while the baby naps can reestablish your relationship.

Investigating Harmony Among Fun and Serious Exercises With A Baby

A presence with another baby is a steady tropical storm of joy and demands. By and by, add to that the commitments of your calling, and you have a certified marketplace showing of rearranging on your hands. It's staggering, yet it's doable, especially with two or three imperative procedures in your device compartment.

Systems for Viable Work-From-Home with a Youngster

Working from home enjoys its benefits, for instance, seeing your young person's most important chuckle. Regardless, it in like manner goes with its piece of hardships, for example, skipping on a call during a crying episode. Spreading out a serious workspace and keeping a set routine can be a help, offering you the valuable chance to switch among work and life as a parent all the more faultlessly.

Improving With Recipe: A Pragmatic Decision

Breastfeeding while simultaneously working all day can be stunningly challenging. If you see that you can't deal with the eventual result of tending to your baby's necessities, upgrading with condition is a practical decision and there's no shame in it. Condition can offer a supportive other choice and facilitate the pressure of making adequate breast milk, allowing you to some degree greater open door and versatility in your schedule.

Benefits of Breastfeeding Your Baby

Thwarting free guts: breastfeeding can diminish the recurrence of the shows to up to 50 percent

Lessening the recurrence of necrotising enterocolitis: this staggering condition in babies has a high loss rate in crippled and less than ideal kids; breastfeeding can diminish its event

Lessening the speed of otitis media: select breastfeeding is connected with a 43% diminishing in otitis media in the underlying 2 years of life.

Confirmation against overweight and chubbiness in later life.

Mental capacity: breastfeeding is positively associated with better execution scores in an extent of information tests.

Reducing the speed of life as a young person illnesses: exclusively breastfeeding at multi week until 4 months could decrease the event of gastrointestinal disorder, lower respiratory package tainting and serous otitis media .

Benefits of Breastfeeding for the Mother

Mothers similarly benefit from breastfeeding their children. These benefits include:

Decreasing possibility of chest infection: a mother's bet of breast threatening development reduces by 4.3% for at customary time frames breastfeeding.

Lessening bet of ovarian sickness: longer breastfeeding is connected with a 30% diminishing peril of ovarian harmful development.

Affirmation against type II diabetes: breastfeeding may offer some protection from diabetes.

Social benefits: these go past the restorative substance of breast milk and integrate enabling maternal responsive approaches to acting; seeing when an infant approaches to acting are prompts for longing and satiety or for comfort and encouragement.

The course of action of breast milk

The essential clinical benefits of breast milk get from its unprecedented synthesis. Breast milk isn't simply a wellspring of enhancements, a living natural fluid . Breast milk involves 87% water, 7% lactose (sugar), 3.8% fat and 1% protein . Together the fat and lactose give around 90% of breast milk's energy content. No matter what the best undertakings of condition producers, no fake feed (which contains 75 sections taking everything into account) has anytime almost imitated breast milk's unpredictability.

The synthesis of breast milk isn't static. It changes after a few times, both during a single feed and over the nursing period, to conform to the changing necessities of your baby's needs . For instance, milk conveyed at every turn in a feed is higher in lactose than later-imparted milk, which is higher in fat. The protein content of breast milk is higher during early start than in the later periods of earliest stages.

The unsaturated fat substance of breast milk is particularly critical in the underlying relatively few weeks after birth, when a newborn child is rapidly coordinating psyche tissue. The impetuses expected to arrange the principal unsaturated fats arachidonic acid and docosahexaenoic acid are not yet totally helpful in the underlying very few extended lengths of life, hence these unsaturated fats ought to be given during dealing with. Docosahexaenoic acid is essential for visual sharpness, cerebrum capacity and improvement.

The most dominating unsaturated fat in breast milk is palmitic acid. Around 70% of palmitic acid is accessible in fats (greasy oils) in an exceptional esterified structure known as SN-2. This is different to the plan of fats contained in infant growth. The SN-2 plan seems to give explicit benefits concerning milder stools, progression of bone prosperity and better assortment in stomach vegetation.

While the piece of breast milk changes considering a mother's eating routine, it remains an area of strength for shockingly its ability to support an infant youngster. Whether or not a mother's own food is modestly poor, her breast milk is most likely going to contain all of the essential enhancements, supplements, minerals, stomach related synthetic substances and synthetics critical to help build up an infant . It will in like manner contain an extent of bioactive parts that can shield against microorganisms, advance safe development and expect a fundamental part in colonizing the infant youngster stomach with an alternate and changed microbiota .The changing making of chest milk similarly adds to the improvement of various and better taste tendencies.

CHAPTER TEN

Looking Forward: Right After Weaning What Is Next?

Breastfeeding reliably arrives at a resolution in the end, each breastfed baby or youngster stops breastfeeding. At times, because of difficulties, breastfeeding your baby arrives at a decision a ton sooner than you thought it would or than you had anticipated. Likewise, with that can come impressions of shock, obligation, sharpness, hurt and dissatisfaction. If you are as of now engaging with breastfeeding completing sooner than you had trusted, we would ask you to chat with someone.

Will Weaning Happen?

What is certain is that all babies quit breastfeeding finally. Kids outgrow breastfeeding in isolation, comparatively as they outgrow other child and little youngster approaches to acting. For certain families, taking on the procedure of being driven by your young person works splendidly and the advancement from breastfeeding to done breastfeeding is standard. It could make all energy less unmistakable, accepting that weaning happens slowly and carefully.

This course of 'typical weaning' allows a baby to make at their own speed, stopping any misrepresentation of breastfeeding as shown by their own standard timing. Rather than picking a specific opportunity to stop breastfeeding, numerous mothers just continue nursing while it is commendable for them and figure out how it ends up. That could mean breastfeeding for a seriously lengthy timespan past what you expected as you first breastfeed your newborn child.

While Weaning Has Happened

Accepting that you are following your child, it is fantastic that they will wean startlingly or at the present moment, especially if they are under one year old. It is genuinely typical for the ordinary weaning cooperation to consume a large portion of the day and feel like several positive developments and two or three back. This can feel frustrating from time to time.

It's typical for youngsters to appear like they are weaning, just to return every now and again with re-energized energy to breastfeed out of the blue or when you thought they had weaned.Another instance is while starting preschool or school, or sickness can habitually provoke a development in breastfeeding when you thought they were ending. That can be unsettling, expecting you are endeavoring to pick in the event that you are at this point breastfeeding or not one day you presumably will not be, and a short time later the accompanying you are again. One mother said: "I thought she was weaning and I was starting to feel the trouble of it about three years old, at this point we are at this point going at four.".

'The Last Breastfeed' most likely won't be a gigantic event. For certain motivations, weaning happens so constantly, that all of a sudden you comprehend your child hasn't mentioned support for quite a while, and you can't recall your last breastfeed - or on the other hand if nothing else, you didn't understand it was the last time.

This is generally speaking the time mothers wish they had gotten more visual memories of their child or youth breastfeeding, not understanding that soon it might be the last breastfeed. Taking photos of you and your child nursing can be really uncommon, so you could have to ponder taking more at this stage.

The subject of what it seems like following weaning isn't examined a ton hence you might be considering whether what you are feeling is run of the mill. It regularly is.

As far as some might be concerned, weaning is an individual change.As breastfeeding arrives at the end it might be an up close and personal time and mothers can experience numerous feelings. For some it might be a time of wretchedness, a sensation of setback for the time that is gone already and a pain that you're one of a kind 'baby days' are passing and behind you. For others it might be a huge assistance and a period you had longed for and thought would never come. Perhaps one second you could feel a freeing impression that the force of breastfeeding is passing and the next second hopeless that this period of life as a parent is drawing in to a close when it has meant a lot to you.

One mother depicted the hour of her child weaning as a bewildering time of feeling a sensation of mishap yet furthermore delight: wretchedness and help. Another, as her child weaned, said that she was completely ready to stop (and was rushed to), but by then recognized it suggested she expected to reconsider how she saw herself as she by and large viewed herself as a breastfeeding mother.

This monstrous mix of sentiments around your breastfeeding adventure arriving at a resolution is typical. Especially in case you tried to get it rolling in bygone times. While breastfeeding has been an especially central piece of how you have mothered your child, it can feel like a new and perhaps uncertain stage.

Inconvenience around weaning is close to 100% the earlier it ends up actually working, or where it happened before you really wanted or had arranged. Where weaning has happened very quickly, mothers can be left with significant vibes of shock, misery, harshness and disappointment. Where weaning has happened unexpectedly, or has been upsetting, in all likelihood, the near and dear impact may be more essential. How old your child is the place where they wean may not be as basic to how you feel about weaning, rather the inclination that things completed well. As Diane Bengson says: "Mothers who wean logically, or who feel that weaning happened when the two they and their young person were ready, as often as possible feel congruity and fulfillment while weaning is done

Nonetheless, whether or not you began weaning or encouraged your child to wean, you could anyway find depictions of pity. Regardless, while weaning is a decent experience for both of you, 'surrendering' can anyway feel near and dear. A couple of mothers and gatekeepers portray it as contemplation for the early times of breastfeeding your baby. Yet again perhaps this is impressively more clear if you understand this is your last baby and you understand you won't be a nursing mother.

Accepting that you felt that your child began weaning instead of you did, and it was sooner than you had expected, that vibe of pity can be more grounded. Then again if your child or more settled kid weaned quickly, you could feel a sensation of hurt or excusal.

Then again you may truly feel just assistance - that you are fulfilled to be forging ahead from the power of bygone times and years and sharing it very well may be said of having your body back. You might feel improved to finally channel your nursing bras and expect to wear articles of clothing that at absolutely no point in the future need straightforward access. You could find a freeing impression that you can plunk down without being drawn nearer to the clinical guardian, and that maybe that unprecedented necessity for you is working with a little and that feels improved.

The key is that anything you are feeling truly about weaning it's by and large anticipated. What one mother experiences won't exactly be comparable to another. Examining it with others (eye to eye or on the web), could help.

HORMONAL CHANGES

It can be genuinely considered common to feel down or rambling - or even deterred - following weaning. Moreover, taking everything into account, the opinions are strong and may mean there is a sensation of anxiety, lack of sleep, shock, swings among high and low perspectives. Somewhat, this is a consequence of hormonal changes happening in your body as you adjust to reducing, and a short time later no more, making milk or having the repeated closeness of your child at your chest. Your chests could regardless continue to make milk, yet leisurely they will stop and for specific mothers it might be quite a while before they can at absolutely no point in the future pound several ways out.

There is little investigation on the point, yet we know that the synthetic compounds so huge in breastfeeding - prolactin (milk making substance) and oxytocin (the substance of fondness and obligated for the milk release reflex) - expect a critical part by they way we feel deep down. Both oxytocin and prolactin add to impressions of calm, love, loosening up, closeness and fulfillment. As breastfeeding closes, both prolactin and oxytocin levels will lower - in this manner may affect your personality and sensation of success. It could last two or three days, or it could occur for longer.

So if you are feeling low or weepy resulting from weaning, it will in general be supporting to understand that in all likelihood, your body is in a manner overseeing hormonal changes, as well as any sentiments you would have around weaning. Whether or not you are totally happy with weaning and acknowledge everything looks great for you both, there are changes happening in your body that could influence how you feel.

It has habitually been depicted as like how you feel hormonally as a part of your female cycle, yet at a similar more exceptional and even more solid. Others could go further and say that they feel really hopeless and deterred for a portion of a month ensuing to weaning. Habitually your synthetics settle inside a portion of a month and you and your child adjust to another musicality where breastfeeding is at absolutely no point in the future piece of your continuous story.

These vibes of pity and general lowness that can happen resulting in weaning are routinely short.

Being fragile and patient with yourself is huge. Expecting you have nonstop low perspective or despairing after the hidden weeks, it may be helpful to chat with your GP. If your child has stopped breastfeeding persistently or they have driven the weaning framework, you could see this as all piece of the groundbreaking strategy of watching your child form into a free minimal person. Your duty of mothering 'your baby' is developing. Perhaps your child is spending longer away from you, may be resting longer or isolated, and maybe there is an inclination that their prerequisite for you isn't precisely so outrageous. That can be both a relief and a change.

You could feel satisfied with how they have created and the sum you have learned about supporting through breastfeeding, yet perhaps can't resist the urge to ponder what it means for you expecting you at absolutely no point in the future have breastfeeding in the picture. Perhaps you are feeling altogether better that your chests are at this point not the mark of intermingling of your child's day?

Where breastfeeding has been basic to you both, it can on occasion have a problematic point of view toward how things could manage without nursing as a go-to or back-up for while supporting is fascinating. How should you get them back to rest if they wake with a horrendous dream around 12 PM? How should you calm them down when the up close and personal tropical storm takes command over them? How might you answer when they thump themselves? How should you get some extra time in bed in the initial segment of the day if your chest no longer offers the desert nursery of calm it once did?

Much of the time looking back at all your breastfeeding relationship gave you and your child, can help with shaping your 'new' picture of sustaining without breastfeeding. Numerous mothers would concur that breastfeeding their youngster past outset is one of their proudest and most unmistakable achievements. Expecting that is what is going on, it could feel right to celebrate or check the event some way or another or one more for you that feels colossal - for both you and your child. Be satisfied!

Additionally, accepting that you are feeling low, or missing that real closeness, now and again finding substitute approaches to partner on a genuine level with your child can help. If your arms are feeling "unfilled" without your child nursing at the chest, cuddling parts, having showers together and playing genuine games with them jumping on you or moving around together, can help with getting a synthetic lift. Fundamental settlement and contact, or sniffing or snuggling your youth's head, can have a significant effect for having a surge of oxytocin.

It's sensible your chests and chest will be an uncommon spot for your child for a long time. Numerous mothers have commented how their more prepared kid truly likes to put their head or hand near their chest, or when upset, will settle into a breastfeeding position without truly breastfeeding.

Looking Forward

As you watch your child wean - be it out and out in isolation, or with some fragile encouragement from you - you could find that you swing between various sentiments and contemplations. Whether weaning passed unexpectedly and feels like a trademark finish to your breastfeeding journey, or you found it a near and dear and testing time, recollecting and perceiving what you achieved and what you have given your child is something you can be appropriately satisfied with.

Breastfeeding has shown you such a lot about seeing your child's necessities and sentiments, their solicitations and their requirements. Your ability to support them, to scrutinize their signs and answer them hasn't changed, yet it might be that rather than offering the chest, you presently address those issues in different ways. Also, remembering that your kid might very well at absolutely no point in the future require comfort at your chest, they really need you.

Numerous mothers and gatekeepers look at their more prepared kids, even grown-up young people, and understand that the condition of their relationship has its foundation back in their nursing days. The closeness, understanding and affiliation that you turned out to be together at the chest all through the long haul, will continue - in new and different ways.

CONCLUSION

Start of Something New!

As our process together closes, recall this: each kick, each restless evening, and each upbeat second has driven you to this wonderful crossroads. Your pregnancy process is extraordinarily yours. As you step into the following part of parenthood, embrace the difficulties, appreciate the triumphs, and confidence in your unbelievable strength. Wishing you perpetual love and bliss on this remarkable experience.

Review Page

Hi Awesome Readers,

We trust "UNDERSTANDING THE PATHWAY OF PREGNANCY" has been a wellspring of help and direction on your remarkable way to parenthood. Your input is unbelievably significant to us! On the off chance that you've partaken in the book, might you at any point kindly pause for a minute to share your considerations in a survey? Your words can help different mothers-to-be find consolation and bits of knowledge inside these pages.

Much obliged to you for being essential for this excursion!

Warm respects

Mikayla Edgell

www.ingramcontent.com/pod-product-compliance
Lightning Source LLC
Chambersburg PA
CBHW070929260726
48661CB00003B/898